I0567936

Dmt

The Complete Simplified Beginners Introductory

(How to Make Dmt Spirit Molecule With a Step-by-step Instructional Guide)

Jayne Olander

Published By **Phil Dawson**

Jayne Olander

Dmt: The Complete Simplified Beginners Introductory (How to Make Dmt Spirit Molecule With a Step-by-step Instructional Guide)

ISBN   978-1-998901-47-0

No part of this guidebook shall be reproduced in any form without permission in writing from the publisher except in the case of brief quotations embodied in critical articles or reviews.

Legal & Disclaimer

The information contained in this ebook is not designed to replace or take the place of any form of medicine or professional medical advice. The information in this ebook has been provided for educational & entertainment purposes only.

The information contained in this book has been compiled from sources deemed reliable, and it is accurate to the best of the Author's knowledge; however, the Author cannot guarantee its accuracy and validity and cannot be held liable for any errors or omissions. Changes are periodically made to this book. You must consult your doctor or get professional medical advice before using

Table Of Contents

Chapter 1: What Is Dimethyltryptamine?

Dimethyltryptamine (DMT) Dimethyltryptamine (DMT), which belongs to the tryptamine family is a psychedelic substance that is found naturally. It is found naturally throughout the human body as well as in some plants. In the human body, DMT is created during normal metabolism by serotonin (a neurotransmitter) and tryptamine-N-methyltransferase (an enzyme). By ingestion, the substance is absorbed, inhaled or inhaled. In nature, DMT can be found in a variety of plant species that belong to genera, such as virola, piptadeniaand mimosa, acacia and many more.

Richard Strassman was one of the first psychologists to research DMT as well as other psychedelic compounds and their effects. He discovered that Dr. Strassman discovered that dimethyltryptamine is released by the pineal gland whenever the person is close to death. This could explain the reason why those who experience near-death experiences frequently have vivid images as well as NDE (near-death experiences) phenomenon. It is interesting to note that the substance is released on day 49 of fetal development. The doctor. Strassman attributes this to the soul's birth. The substance is commonly described as the "spirit chemical" or "God molecules."

Uses of DMT

In various varieties, numerous ethnic tribes and cultures throughout the world especially in South America, use dimethyltryptamine. In the context of cultural ceremonies ethnic tribes utilize DMT in order to feel spiritually connected to God. South American tribes inhale and consume Yopo (anadenanthera peregrina) which is a plant that contains an abundance of DMT. Inhaling or ingestion of the drug can cause people to experience psychedelic experiences.

Amazonian Amerindian tribes also ingest the chemical by inhaling Ayahuasca (an intoxicant brew) to heal and for divination reasons. The United States, many people make use of bongs and vaporizers to breathe in DMT. The effects of DMT last just a few minutes however the "high" that one feels when drinking DMT is completely altered by the state and is regarded as to be intense.

Dangers and Effects of DMT

In simple terms If taken in large quantities and uncontrolled, dimethyltryptamine may cause serious health problems. The users of DMT may fall into a coma-like state or attain an unconscious state. In many cases, those who are unconscious be vomiting, which can lead to choke and even death.

In moderate doses The various effects of DMT can include increased body temperature, an increase in heart rate, irritation to the lung terrifying fear stomach pain as well as a change in the perception of time, as well as intense visual psychedelics. Other effects could include visions and sensations of movement or time slowing or increasing speed. Colors can become blurred and people may have double vision.

The Law

In several countries, dimethyltryptamine can be classified as a Class A (or Schedule I drug. It is unlawful to own, sell or offer to anyone else. If you are found to be in possession of DMT the maximum penalty is seven years of jail and/or a huge fine. Even if one gives or distributes DMT even to friends it is possible to end up in prison for the rest of their lives or, at most, paying a large fine.

If a person is questioned by the police for taking or having DMT The police will usually decide to take action, which could include an official caution or a criminal prosecution or an arrest. It is a serious matter should one be found guilty of an offense involving drugs. It could hinder individuals from traveling to any other country and the types of jobs that one could be considered for are limited. It is also unlawful to drive if one is intoxicated by DMT.

Taking DMT

The substance isn't orally active when it is combined with an MAOI (monoamine inhibits oxidase) such as the ones in harmala alkaloids. They are created by plants, such as the ayahuasca plant (Banisteriopsis caapi) and Syrian rue (Peganum harmala). Within the body of the individual, and without an inhibitor monoamine oxidase quickly breaks down DMT that was orally taken in and leads insignificant psychoactive effect. In its purest form, DMT is normally smoked or inhaled.

Chapter 2: History of Dimethyltryptamine

in 1931 Richard Manske attempted to synthesize dimethyltryptamine in a massive period of chemical experiments in the wake of the discovery of mescaline towards the close in the late 19th century. In the 19th century the effects of DMT on human consciousness or its use within South American tribal concoctions were recognized, and DMT was largely ignored until about a decade later when South American shamans' potions and concoctions became the object of intense interest within the burgeoning area of psychopharmacology.

In his 1946 paper written in Spanish, O. Goncalves first isolated dimethyltryptamine in M. Teniflora (Mimosa hostilis). Following that, further research of South American shamans' plants led to DMT being isolated in the two species, P. Peregrina and Piptadenia macrocarpa. That was in 1955. Despite its widespread usage by tribes of culture throughout South America, the general public was not aware of the psychoactive effects of DMT till Stephen Szara reported it in 1956.

Szara is the Hungarian psychotherapist and chemist who worked in the shadow of the Iron Curtain, was unable to get mescaline and LSD through Sandoz. Therefore, he developed one of his own DMT after reading about the presence of the substance within South American shamans' plants. He then hoped the substance would exhibit "psychedelic" properties of the DMT he had synthesized.

After several failed doses of oral medication Szara came to the conclusion that an enzyme in the gastrointestinal system or substance could be neutralizing dimethyltryptamine. Szara was the first to study DMT's psychoactive properties by injecting the substance synthesized. The results of his research would eventually be made public dimethyltryptamine's properties to the world.

Soon after, Szara and his DMT stash fled Hungary and then relocated towards in the U.S. where he found employment at Bethesda Maryland's National Institutes of Health. He was employed there for over 30 years. When he retired in 1991, Szara was the National Institute on Drug Abuse's Director for Preclinical Research.

Illegal Substance

In 1966, dimethyltryptamine became classified as illegal following the time it was made available to the new psychedelic underground via the correspondence between Ralph Metzner, Timothy Leary along with William S.

Burroughs. Burroughs had wrote in his correspondence with Leary that DMT could be dangerous to experiment with after he nearly overdosed self-injecting the drug in London in the year 1960.

Nick Sands is credited as discovering that DMT could be smoked in which case the discovery briefly led to the rise of DMT's popularity in underground users. It was in 1968 that Agurell, Lindgren, and Holmstedt first realized that the effects of ayahuasca could be due to the interaction of natural DMT as well as monoamine oxidase inhibitors.

In the year 1970 in the year 1970, The United States Congress approved the "Scheduling Laws" that made it virtually impossible to study DMT, LSD, and mescaline within the United States. The law stopped scientific research into DMT in the United States until the FDA-approved clinical trials conducted by Rick

Strassman at the University of New Mexico. The trials ran from 1990 until 1995.

Although DMT was (and remains) prohibited throughout the United States, other international governments have allowed its use in a limited degree and research into DMT was conducted internationally. The possibility that dimethyltryptamine may be a human-specific endogenous substance first became apparent when scientists found DMT in the brains of rats as well as mice's brains. In 1965 an German team announced that they had extracted DMT via human blood.

The year 1972 was when Julian Axelrod discovered that DMT was detected in the human brain. Then, he discovered DMT in urine of humans and in the fluid (cerebrospinal) that covers and surrounds the brain. When the mechanisms by the body produced DMT were discovered it was declared to be the first exogenous human psychoactive. It was in 1965 that S. T. Christian discovered 5-MeO-DMT found in the cerebrospinal liquid.

Chapter 3: The Science Behind DMT

DMT (dimethyltryptamine) is a member of the tryptamine compound family that comprises of biologically-active compounds, including neurotransmitters such as the main pineal hormone and 5-hydroxytryptamine (serotonin), entheogens and melatonin, including DMT, 5-HO-DMT (bufotenine), O-phosophoryl-4-HO-DMT (psilocybin), and 5-methoxy-dimethyltryptamine (5-MeO-DMT). Each of these compounds has the same indole-ring structure which means that the backbone of the indole can be considered to be a component in the constitution of complex entheogens such as ibogaine as well as LSD.

The Indole Ring

Although magic mushrooms (psilocybin) and LSD are among the most popular psychedelic psychedelics, the most interesting tryptamines are the entheogens that originate from the body, such as 5-MeO and DMT. Why are they so fascinating? This is because the two entheogens do not have to be laboratory-manufactured nor are they extracted from a toad's venom or a plant. They are created in our bodies. Since they are endogenous, this means they are a component of the human body, just as hair, bones or teeth are a part of the human body.

Since DMT and 5-MeO have the same features as neurotransmitters. They can both cross the blood-brain-synthetic barrier and allow them to have a profound influence on consciousness of the human. DMT is particularly unique because it is considered to be an "brain hormone."

Neurotransmitters and Endorphins

Although they may affect the perception of consciousness and spirituality, dimethyltryptamine as well as 5-MeO are two of the entheogens naturally created in the body of a human. The body also has the capacity to make other popular "drugs" like endorphins that are morphine-like substances.

Finding endorphins inside our bodies was thought to be an important scientific breakthrough and the scientists who discovered endorphins for their efforts were given the Nobel Prize. Many people would believe that finding the natural production of entheogens could have been regarded as equally significant. However, due to strictures imposed on psychedelics that were already known during the 70s, studies into the entheogens was halted and the progress of research was slowed.

The research on psychedelics known to exist like LSD and psilocybin have increased in recent years especially in relation to their claimed medical advantages. In the end, however, U.S. Drug Enforcement Agency authorized only one study regarding DMT. The study mentioned above was the University of New Mexico study which was conducted by Dr. Strassman between 1990 and 1995.

The Most Basic Tryptamine Psychedelic

Of all the psychedelics that contain tryptamine, DMT is the simplest. Dimethyltryptamine, when compared with other molecules is small , and weighs around 188 molecular units. It is not that much bigger than glucose as it is the simplest of all sugars within the body. The weight of glucose is 180 molecular units and has a weight 10x greater than water molecules (18 molecular units). As a reference the weights for the other substances that are psychoactive are mescaline 211 molecular units as well as 323 molecular units of LSD.

Dimethyltryptamine can be described as a close to serotonin and its chemical properties are similar to those of other psychedelics that are well-known. DMT alters the serotonin receptors in a similar way like mescaline psilocybin and LSD. Serotonin receptors are found all over the body , and are found in the glands, skin muscles, as well as blood vessels.

The brain is where dimethyltryptamine can exert its most powerful effects. The brain's regions that are rich in serotonin receptors that are sensitive to DMT are involved in thinking and perception as well as mood. Although the brain restricts access to a variety of chemicals and substances and chemicals, the brain has an "special interest" in the area of DMT.

Additionally, a highly sensitive organ such as the brain is prone to imbalances in metabolism and the toxins. The blood-brain barrier, an invisible barrier that can't be broken, stops "unwelcome" elements from exiting the bloodstream and moving into the brain tissues through the capillaries' walls. This defense also blocks fats and complex carbohydrates other tissues use for energy. In contrast, it uses glucose as the purest form of fuel.

Certain molecules are able to undergo active transport across the blood brain barrier. Certain molecules are specially designed to transport their contents to brains, the process that takes an enormous amount of energy. It is obvious the reason why, in a lot of cases the brain is able to transport certain chemicals to its surroundings. For instance amino acids essential to maintain the protein level within the brain may be transported into the brain.

In recent times, DMT has enjoyed resurgence in the popular consciousness. It is hoped that more research of a positive nature is conducted on dimethyltryptamine as well as 5-MeO-DMT's distinctive properties.

Chapter 4: The Effects of DMT

The limitations on dimethyltryptamine use and distribution differ from country to country. In accordance with the international laws, DMT can be classified as an Schedule I drug under the United Nations' 1971 Convention on Psychotropic Substances which means that the use of DMT is intended to be limited to scientific research and medical purposes. However, natural substances containing DMT (like Ayahuasca) are not subject to regulation by the Psychotropic Convention.

In general, DMT is not addictive. A study of ritual-based users of ayahuasca revealed that "A mix of harmala alkaloids as well as DMT that is used for religious purposes is safe in a manner equivalent to mescaline, methadone or codeine. The potential for dependence of oral DMT and the risks of long-term psychological distress are quite low.

The Dr. Rick Strassman has recorded some of the physical effects of DMT. In his "Dose-response study of N,N-dimethyltryptamine in humans," Strassman recorded that a moderate dose of DMT led to a slightly-elevated heart rate, blood pressure, rectal pleasure, and pupil diameter. This was in addition to a rise in blood levels of beta-endorphin, corticotropin, prolactin, as well as cortisol. When he conducted Strassman's DMT research, Strassman noted that growth hormone levels in blood also increased when exposed to DMT doses. Unaffected were melatonin doses.

DMT isn't as addicting as heroin, alcohol, or cocaine, since dimethyltryptamine doesn't trigger similar addiction-seeking behavior. Similar to addictive substances, however, DMT produces increased tolerance for certain people who regularly consume the substance. Users then have to take larger DMT doses to attain the effects they have experienced previously due to their heightened tolerance.

Dimethyltryptamine is usually consumed by smoking, inhaling or snorted, and the effects of it are known as"trips. "trip," which typically lasts between 45 minutes to 1 hour. As we mentioned previously in the past, when consumed orally, DMT does not have any effect when it is not combined with other substances. If taken excessively, DMT also comes with its own risks. It may cause irrational judgement that can cause accidents and reckless decisions. In excess, it can cause terrifying flashbacks or even trips.

Major Effects of Dimethyltryptamine

It is known that there aren't any lasting adverse effects from dimethyltryptamine because the effects of consuming the drug last, up to an hour. The psychedelic experiences experienced by taking the drug are mostly determined by the user's subconscious mind. Dimethyltryptamine could be harmful, especially for those who have experienced mental health issues prior to. It is not uncommon of for users to suffer an unpleasant experience and then end up hurting themselves in a anxiety.

Users may experience auditory as well as visual hallucinations. It could even result in the sensation of euphoria. DMT could alter the perception of the speed of time. In this case, time appears to be moving slower or speeding up. In this case it is typical that pupils dilate. For the effects on the eyes many users agree that it's difficult to explain what you see to a person who is not familiar using the drug.

Because DMT is a risk for those who have an history of mental health issues It can also be dangerous for those who are with a fearful or stressed state. DMT can cause the onset of undiscovered or lingering mental health issues for certain users. For certain people, the anxieties and fears are amplified when traveling. It can be a frightening and terrifying experience, which is often accompanied by vomiting and nausea.

Users who use indiscriminately DMT have been reported to inflict harm on the public and themselves. In these instances there is a chance of suicide. If a person is going through the motions, there isn't a option to end the journey until the effects decrease. This is the reason it is suggested by the users to always keep an sober person with them when you decide to test DMT in particular when you are first trying it. There are some reports of negative effects of taking DMT as well, flashbacks of bad experiences have been reported by a few users, even after the effects of the drug have faded.

Psychological Side Effects of Taking DMT

Apart from the physical consequences of taking dimethyltryptamine the psychological side effects are often unpleasant for those who do not know how to correctly dosage or consume DMT. A few of these psychological side effects could include emotional disturbances, depersonalization real-life hallucinations, as well as spiritual panic.

Spiritual Emergency

In the event of a spiritual crisis the psychological consequences that come from DMT as well as other psychoactive substances can be a source of anxiety. As per psychologist David Lukoff, such experiences could trigger shifts in the nature of reality, that can trigger anxiety and fear. An abrupt change or loss in meaning is known as an issue with the spiritual or religious realm and is often called spiritual emergency.

In particular, ceremonies involving ayahuasca can help with these sometimes painful situations in a shamanic context of a particular culture through the combination of DMT-containing drugs along with other rituals, such as the chanting. The tourism industry based on ayahuasca, that is growing in popularity, doesn't always help those who experience mental instability outside of the ritual's boundaries.

Realistic Hallucinations

If it's about real hallucinations, people who use psychedelics typically know what hallucinations feel aren't real because they are a combination of the senses. But with DMT the knowledge of this kind does not have to be present. Because of the effects of dissociation users may experience the sensation of being in another dimension or an alternate reality that is more vivid and compelling than dreams or waking awareness. As per the Office of Diversion Control, there are a few DMT users who have reported altered body image as well as real auditory hallucinations.

Emotional Disturbances

In the presence of DMT, many users might feel relaxed. Some users experience fear and anxiety in particular if they're uncomfortable with losing control at the most intense stage. In a study from 1994 co-authored by Rick Strassman there were cases of individuals who had taken psychoactive drugs who felt that euphoria was present or alternating with anxiety. Similar to other tryptamines DMT is not associated to addiction.

Depersonalization

Dimethyltryptamine, as well as other substances that contain tryptamine, like psilopcybe fungi could cause modifications in how people identify themselves. Dimethyltryptamine's metabolism is rapid and it peaks in just 90 seconds. The resulting psychological shifts are what are what the U.S. Drug Enforcement Agency has described as the "businessman's journey." A complete disappearance of identity and self with objects that are not real and cause users to be able to feel deeply contemplation of their own existence.

Signs of Addiction and Treatment

Although it isn't addictive in itself However, the repeated usage of DMT can result in psychological dependence. It is when a person gets a buzz from the drug such that he or is convinced that they will no be able to function without it. Someone who uses DMT who is on a high is very obvious, since they can sense or perceive things that aren't true. One indication that an individual is psychologically addicted to DMT is when they exhibit irrational behavior that the user is exhibiting.

DMT does not count as a drug that is used in social settings It is a potential sign of DMT misuse is spending longer in solitude without responding other people. The presence of dangerous materials and equipment for chemistry could indicate that someone is producing DMT for commercial or personal reasons.

One of the best ways to stop the negative effects of DMT is to participate in activities that aren't associated with drugs. Although the effects of DMT are severe however, theoretically it's simpler to stop using it completely. Although recovering from the effects of a DMT addiction shouldn't require excessive medical attention however, it is advisable to seek advice from an expert for guidance in dealing with any potential psychological cravings that might arise.

Chapter 5: Pros and Cons of DMT

The line that separates the positive between dimethyltryptamine's positive and negative aspects are slightly blurred, with DMT being classified as a Schedule I controlled or Grade A chemical when it is it is manufactured in a laboratory and an unregulated chemical when it occurs naturally in certain plants. The main problem with DMT is the legalization process, where both the negative and positive sides are presented with their respective aspects.

The side that supports dimethyltryptamine's legalization has a number of positive points. Over the past several centuries, DMT has been used in a variety of South American cultures as a tool to perform rites of passageor a sacrament or for worship. The regulation of the drug in some countries has prevented individuals from observing their faith. Furthermore, its psychedelic properties have been examined in relation to revealing one's own self and assisting in the fight against powerful psychological processes such as addiction. Furthermore, the claim the dimethyltryptamine effect is "natural" because it's produced by the brain makes the notion that it is a good idea to boost the amount naturally in the human body, like how we supplement their bodies with exogenous hormones.

The people who oppose legalization of DMT have valid arguments. The drug is hallucinogenic and if used improperly, DMT can lead to the danger of self as well as to others. Additionally the MAOI (monoamine oxidase inhibitor) is required to make the drug efficient in brewing drinks for oral consumption with DMT. If misused, MAOIs can seriously harm the individual and a negative trip can psychologically mark the person for a long period of time. There are studies suggesting that overdosing or prolonged DMT use can be linked to schizophrenia.

Near-Death Experience

As previously mentioned dimethyltryptamine, a compound has been linked to what's described as"near-death experiences. "near-death sensation." In the quest to solve the near-death experience mystery, scientists have suggested several theories about possible reasons. One theory is that of Carl Sagan's theory through oxygen deprivationtheories, neurochemical theories and psychological dissociation. In the realm of neurochemical theories, psychoactive substances such as DMT and ketamine are involved.

The author, the Dr. Rick Strassman's work DMT The Spirit Molecule, suggested that after death the pineal tissue begins to decay could release dimethyltryptamine directly into spinal fluid. This gives the brain's emotional as well as sensory centers to generate an awareness that remains. D.R. Hill as well as Michael Persinger have also conjectured that all kinds of spiritual experiences (NDEs including) may be related to events which trigger the release of DMT through the pineal gland. Pim van Lommel is an NDE researcher is a writer on the parallels between NDE and DMT trips.

There are other people who deny the role of DMT in NDEs. The Methodist university's Dr. Michael Potts compared the DMT experience's elements to aspects of NDE that are in the "NDE Scale" that was developed in the late the Dr. Bruce Greyson. Based on Dr. Potts, key or common NDE phenomenon have not been documented by DMT users, such as travelling through a tunnel in order to enter another dimension. According to him, the permanent changes following a NDE appear to be the norm and not an only exception. However, the permanent changes that occur after DMT experiences are more of an exception than a norm. Additionally, Potts suggests that DMT isn't the only thing which causes the appearance of NDEs.

The Most Powerful Psychedelic

Dimethyltryptamine is regarded as the most potent psychedelic known to the human race. It's difficult to ask researchers to explain their DMT experience since the majority of cases are extremely intense. Furthermore, they can be too complicated to comprehend when you are who are not familiar with the experience of tripping. In addition, a trip on dimethyltryptamine is extremely fast-growing and has just a few minutes (one hour or less) however, the experience will vary significantly based on the person who is taking it regardless of whether the location is the same (unlike many psychoactives).

Chapter 6: DMT Compared to Similar Substances

Since dimethyltryptamine is an hallucinogenic chemical that is comparable to, and frequently compared to substances such as psilocybin and peyote or ayahuasca. LSD. These hallucinogens all produce altering perceptions by acting on neurons in the brain which make use of serotonin (a neurotransmitter). Particularly, the most significant effects are felt in the prefrontal cortex of the brain and other brain regions that are essential in regulating arousal and psychological responses to stress and anxiety.

The short-term effects of different psychoactive compounds are likely to differ significantly. In LSD there are a few effects include dizziness and sleepiness. There is also the possibility of dry mouth, sweating and a loss of appetite. LSD also raises the body's temperature, blood pressure as well as heart rates. It can cause the sensation of tremors, weakness and the sensation of numbness. People who use LSD may also experience intense emotional shifts as well as bouts of insanity. These shifts could range from joy to anxiety. Some of these shifts are so fast that the user may experience many different emotions simultaneously.

Peyote is an naturally occurring substance and can be found within a specific cactus that is native in Mexico which is grown in some parts of Texas. It is a controlled substance that, although but not as strict as DMT. If used in excess peyote could cause excessive sweating, flushing ataxia, incoordination, as well as increased body temperature and heart rate.

Psilocybin can be found in the form of what's often called "magic mushrooms."

When you take this psychedelic, people are able to experience relaxation (a similar feeling when taking marijuana in small amounts). Users can also experience spiritual/introspective experiences coupled with panic attacks, paranoia, and nervousness. But, misidentification of poisonous mushrooms that appear like psilocybin could result in fatal, but inadvertent poisoning.

For DMT The results include increased blood pressure, hallucinations which always are triggered by altered environments along with the body's spatial and physical distortions. In the form of a component of DMT, ayahuasca may result in increased blood pressure and vomiting that is caused by tea. While taking ayahuasca, one may also experience a state of altered consciousness and visions that are not your normal.

Effects of Hallucinogens

They can be manufactured or naturally extracted from cacti or other mushrooms or naturally produced in the body of humans, hallucinogens when consumed in excess, can cause a variety of intense and potentially hazardous negative effects.

When they are consumed, hallucinogens can cause people to experience sounds, images, and experience feelings that are not real however seem real in the time. Hallucinogen's effects usually occur between 20 and 90 minutes after the ingestion, and last up to 12 hours.

In general the experiences aren't always predictable and differ from person to individual. Therefore, regardless of their source and whether they're manufactured or naturally occurring hallucinogens' effects are remarkably alike. They may harm your health if consumed in excess.

Chapter 7: The Future of Dimethyltryptamine

In the same way that as Dr. Rick Strassman is one of the most prominent researchers in DMT and researchers, he is planning to pursue his DMT research at the New Mexico Cottonwood Research Foundation. While he is there researcher Dr. Steven Barker of Louisiana State University is working on an ultra-sensitive method to measure dimethyltryptamine that naturally occurs inside the human body. Strassman and Barker are looking to compare the normal levels of dimethyltryptamine with those found in altered state in clinical conditions.

Strassman along with his group want to design a new paradigm for Western consciousness research. The team is hoping to study the many different forms of human consciousness as well as their biochemical, psychological and genetic causes. They want to determine the most effective way to use these states in increasing wisdom and creativity as well as healing.

Ayahuasca

The interest in the ayahuasca plant, which has DMT is definitely increasing. In the continuous Global Drug Survey, Adam Winstock is a researcher and co-authors discovered the fact that DMT "had the highest number of users" in comparison to other psychoactive substances, including ketamine LSD and magical mushrooms.

The results of the Winstock survey are confirmed by the National Survey on Drug Use and Health. Both surveys' data showed that the amount of DMT users in the United States has been steadily growing since 2006, ranging from 688,000 in 2006 to 1,475,000 by 2012. The survey also showed that the most recent DMT users are more likely to be men who were still in school and younger.

The Global Drug Survey, which is held every year, offers an insight into how the use of drugs by users. Since the survey doesn't use random sampling, it's not able to pinpoint the frequency of a specific drug's use. However, it can detect some of the most significant trends.

As per one L.A. Weekly report, Los Angeles has at least three subcommittees for ayahuasca which are in operation. At any given time within New York City, there are between 50 and 100 ceremonies using dimethyltryptamine to make the form of ayahuasca.

At the beginning of the millennium people who couldn't discover "acid" within their towns began to fly across the world to Brazil, Ecuador, or Peru. They hoped to experience the currently obscure ayahuasca experiences. In an interview with the novel This is Your Country on Drugs A Peruvian shaman (who was seeking anonymity) stated that prior to 2001, he had never seen an American attend his ceremonies.

Psychedelic Tourism

This type of psychedelic travel quickly gained popularity and Ayahuasca tours are now available across South American countries that have no customary or religious tradition of drinking the drink. Tommy Thomas, a Costa Rican farmer, also commented about the current trend on This is Your Country on Drugs.

Formerly , a Washington D.C-based property developer Thomas has relocated to Costa Rica over 20 years ago to make a living by growing as well as cultivating plants that produce hallucinogenic effects.

At the time his hallucinogenic plants did not yield a profit, and he shifted to cultivating traditional crops. He did notice an increase in the sales of hallucinogenic plants starting in 2005.

One sign that ayahuasca tourism has seen a dramatic increase in coverage through the media. Newspapers such as National Geographic have run stories about the writer's South American excursions with nausea, mosquito-strewn camps as well as boat, plane and bus journeys. But, there's really no reason for Americans to go in South America to experience an Ayahuasca-based trip.

The unidentified Peruvian shaman offered his ayahuasca-infused brew to countries such as India, Italy, and Spain in the 90s. He didn't introduce his brew into the United States because he did not believe that Americans would take it seriously. Then, he came across some Americans who made him feel welcome into San Francisco. Today, he travels back to America frequently. United States often, and says that there are numerous cities and towns who want for him to move to the United States.

My Path to DMT

Have you ever considered the three most important questions? What are we born from what are we, who are we and what's the purpose of our existence? I've been thinking about these things throughout my entire existence ... It began when my father gifted me a book on my birthday. It stated, "Everything I'd like to learn about". The book contains 150 pages, however there was just one subject I was interested in back then the world of our universe.Although I wasn't in a position to read I did look at the chapter many times, when I finally began the book, I was astonished. My mom bought the book another time, as it was not readable anymore because it had been worn out over time. I still have the book to this day and I'm convinced that the universe was created in this book or perhaps later ...

It was 2011 when I started my own business as a web designer , and finally found time to work with things which were close to my heart. So I began to read about subjects that truly interested me.

Metaphorically, I took in every bit of information I could. Particularly interesting was the subject "The reality of us".

As time went by, I was exposed to concepts like the astral plane, mental dimension multiverses, etc. In the end I came to an age where I needed to put my knowledge to the test.

While I was a believer in a lot of it, it's only the beginning of understanding and the naive belief in something that is not backed by any solid proof could not satisfy my ardent curiosity. It was my desire to find out if the mind exists outside of the body, and whether there's anything else beyond our materialistic reality.

Therefore, I began the practice of transcendental meditation and employed the methods described within the texts. My experience was not great. Even though I had number of positive experiences, after several months of intensive practice, I didn't really make the breakthrough. I was ready to give up when, on chance, I ran into another old acquaintance I had not visited for over two years. He shared with me an upcoming film that explains the way people go away from their bodies following the use of an odd substance known as DMT. I was stunned when he mentioned it and, somehow, I knew that this was the reason behind my responses.

So, I started to research DMT and with every piece I read I discovered many interesting facts and discovered many connections to other subjects for instance. for instance. the importance in the pineal gland or the connection with dreams and near-death experience, or the connection to a variety of religions and ancient civilizations. The thought was , "That isn't possible How could we have overlooked the connection for all this time!", And my desire to investigate it increased to the point that it shook me to the inside. There was no other option and I needed to figure out how to obtain DMT. I found it, and in the next chapters, I will provide you with the details I needed in the past.

I give the most importance to the transformation of consciousness. For the entire development of humanity is a shift and expanding of consciousness. The whole process of cultural and other growth depends on it. -Albert Hofmann- (discoverer of LSD)

What is DMT?

At first glance, N-N-dimethyltryptamine ($C_{12}H_{16}N_2$), abbreviated as DMT, is an endogenous neurotransmitter from the tryptamine family, which was produced synthetically in the laboratory first in 1931 by R.H.F. Manske. Manske was discovered to be an organic substance by the late 1950s. It is present in a variety of species of plants, which makes DMT one of the most alkaloid (indole alkaloid). In later times, the substance was discovered in various animals and humans. Even though DMT is made in our bodies however, it is thought to be the most powerful psychedelic drug known to humans.

Our body is also home to various tryptamine alkaloids, like serotonin, a neurotransmitter. Serotonin is a kind of tryptamine commonly referred to as 5-hydroxytryptamine. Its chemical structure DMT shares interesting similarities with serotonin and Psilocin. Psilocin is a highly psychoactive substance that is also a variant of DMT known as 4-OH-DMT. is a secret among the general public.

Chemical structures of serotonin, psilocin, and N-N-dimethyltryptamine

In comparison to other molecules, DMT is rather tiny. Its weight is 188,molecular units'. This implies that it is not as big as glucose, which is the most common sugar we have in our bodies and weighs only around 180 molecular units.

It is hard to identify DMT within the body of a human since it is quickly activated by an enzyme known as monoamine oxide (MAO).

But, research suggests that human DMT is created in the pineal gland. One proof could be the fact that DMT was found inside the glands that produce pineal hormones in rabbits back in 2013. However, other organs can be considered to be the supply of the endogenous DMT and.

A simplified figure of tryptamine Synthesis

Dr. Rick Strassman believes that the release of DMT is increased at the time of birthday, our death when we sleep, and during difficult events. Particularly talked about is the function that DMT during dreams. There is even a belief to be that the release DMT may be the neurological underlying factor for the sensation of dreaming.

In this regard there is a specific role for shamanic experiences. the shamanic experience and meditation is extremely likely.

Shamans from the Amazon region have their own unique version that they use for DMT consumption. They created a DMT-containing drink known as Ayahuasca.

In normal circumstances, DMT does not have any effects when taken orally, since, as stated, it is instantly removed via the enzyme (MAO).

The shamans discovered the plant (Banisteriopsis caapi) that blocks the MAO which means that the powerful psychedelic effect of DMT may be felt when you ingest it. The archaeological finds in Ecuador indicate the existence of indigenous peoples performing Ayahuasca ceremonies for more than five thousand years.

But, DMT is also transformed into a smokeable form that produces a heightened mind-altering sensation.

Subjects have reported on alternate reality with different physical laws where contact with alien living beings can be possible.

This sensation lasts less than 15 minutes, but the duration of experience is usually to be much longer.

DMT is strictly forbidden in most countries. This means that everyone is constantly carrying prohibited substances around in their bodies that is quite absurd!

DMT - The Spirit Molecule

Professor. Rick Strassman conducted state-approved clinical research at the University of New Mexico from 1990 until 1995. He involved sixty participants who were experienced with psychedelics. All received around 400 doses of DMT intravenously. The events were documented with remarkable detail, where participants often described encounters with intelligent non-human beings. Most of them believed they had the most profound experiences they have had in their life.

The book supports the assertion that it is natural to release DMT in the pineal gland facilitates the soul's movement through and out of the body, and is a part of the experience of death and birth. Even in the most profound states of meditation as well as in sexual experience that transcendent It is evident that it is in some way.

If used with care, DMT could usher in an extraordinary period of advances in the research of some of the most fascinating mystical and mysterious regions of the human psyche as well as its spirituality. [1]

Strassman's amazing research was released in the month of December in DMT the Spirit Molecule. The book was published in 12 different languages, and sold in excess of 100,000 copies.

In addition to the book, there's an accompanying documentary with the same title that is available to view on YouTube.

The film and book are extremely thrilling and contain facts that should not be located online. The reports in particular completely blew my mind.

Is the Consumption of DMT Dangerous?

The feeling that surrounds you after taking DMT is that of being struck by lightning bolts that are noetic. The normal world is changed in a flash and not with a single hallucination. It is an experience that is so alien to you is its extreme astonishment. Nothing will be able to prepare you for the experiences that flood your mind when you step into this world.

The remarkable speed of the experiment suggests that it's very safe. It is virtually eliminated out of the body in ten minutes. It is a paradox it is that DMT is the most powerful and safest of all. This is probably due to the fact that there are reasons not revealed to the public, DMT occurs in normal brain metabolism. -Terence McKenna-

Physical dangers

While DMT is among the most powerful psychedelic drugs but it's also one of the most secure. Because the human body already contains trace amounts of DMT The brain understands precisely how to deal with it, and it can also metabolize the substance with ease.

It is at this point that we must make one must be aware that, although DMT and LSD molecules are similar in chemical composition, DMT as well as LSD molecules are quite similar in chemical structure, LSD is an alien substance that, when consumed causes damage to neurons in the brain. DMT is constantly transported across the blood-brain-barrier throughout the body. This is an extremely rare event due to the fact that the blood-brain-barrier acts as an inbuilt filter that is used to isolate your brain from bloodstream. The nature of the fact that DMT can traverse the blood-brain-barrier without restriction confirms the absurdity of this chemical.

In reality it is possible to say that DMT is among the most safe psychedelics however it is certainly safer than cigarettes and alcohol.

Mental/ spiritual dangers:

DMT is a powerful impact on the mind, which is not to be ignored. A few of the smallest risks that may be experienced result from inadequate preparation.

Every person should consider that DMT is able to change your thinking, which can result in you not being able to integrate the experience into your daily life, leading to unexpected consequences for your future. It is beneficial to get some experience in the state of psychedelic consciousness prior to beginning an DMT journey.

Setting and setting (inner mental state and the external environment) can play a significant aspect in how you deal with the event.

What do Psychedelic Substances Cause in the Brain

There aren't exact studies on the brain's reaction to DMT intoxication, however there has been some research regarding how psilocybin affects the brain. as well as

LSD that are like their chemical structures of DMT. Additionally the three substances are extremely similar to the endogenous neurotransmitter, serotonin, and mimic its effects. This implies that they are able to are able to bind to specific receptors for serotonin, providing the same signalling to the nerve cell. Because not all, but only a narrow selection of serotonin receptors get activated (in particular, 5-HT1A, 5-HT2A and 5-HT2C receptors through LSD along with 5-HT2A receptors and 5-HT2C via psilocybin) The processing of information happens inside the brain. [1]

By activation of specific serotonin receptors, information-processing parts of the brain are opened, resulting in a large increase in impulse transmission. After that, the sensory information cannot be being compared to information stored in memory and is no longer taken as normal. This could result in a totally altered ego and experience of the environment. When there is a high levels of activation of serotonin receptors that only single, distinct and unrelated pictures are processed. [1]

Many people experience this phenomena as a remarkably moving whole, accompanied by an inner stream of visions.

LSD as well as magic mushrooms stimulate serotonin receptors, without the requirement in nerve cells for release of serotonin like the ecstasy (MDMA). So, there is no serotonin deficiency that could trigger depression after a psychedelic trip, is something to be worried about. [1]

USuppression of Spirituality

Why are Psychedelics Forbidden?

What happens when you discover that you've lived in a dream since the day you were born, and the reality actually is very different?

Do you find it annoying that you spent a lot of your life within an illusion, not knowing the full extent of the world around you?

What would your life be like been if you'd been aware of that prior to now?

These are all pure philosophical, but maybe they can be connected to our daily lives.

What do you consider to be the truth? Are you able to say it's what you already know? If yes then, the truth is an entirely subjective thing which is unique for each person, since every person has different experiences throughout our lives, according to the is the culture or region of the globe we are born into.

In this instance: majority of Germans believe that

The Amazon natives eat ayahuasca to be an intoxicant (if they've had heard of it prior to) However, the indigenous people of the Amazon are aware that ayahuasca is used to heal information, harmony, and healing. This is the way that perception and reality is different! Anyone who has been taught something from the time of birth, doesn't question the truth of it, they accept it as a given and it's difficult for him to change this habitual belief system, as it has become part of his unconscious.

Therefore, when drugs, or bad tongues refer to them as narcotics, are always depicted as negative, the negative attitude towards related subjects is already pre-programmed or, more accurately or programmed within.

What are the reasons psychedelics are so dangerous?

Psychedelics are able to alter the meanings and patterns that you have cultivated in your environment. give you a new perspective of your place with the Universe, obtain greater insights that may alter your life in the past.

The short version is that psychedelics possess the capacity to broaden the boundaries of perception and let you think beyond the norm.

Why are they not allowed? It's great to know more about the world around us. It's almost as if we don't need to discover more about the world to keep in our traditional ways.

What should a person find out that his cancer could be treated with an natural, unpatented medication? (I don't offer any guarantee of any sort of salvation here)

Do you think he'd still visit the doctor to undergo chemotherapy?

Perhaps probably not! How would society like if it hadn't been taught to be a godly saint? It's probably not like ours!

It would be totally different!

What could happen if psychedelics became legal? Society, as we know ittoday, could not exist in absolute certainty. It would be a community that is committed to nature which does not consider itself as an independent entity with the all of the planet, instead, rather as an integral part of the whole that is small, but extremely significant.

They aren't illegal because an obedient government is worried that you could fall from a third-story window. They are unlawful since they disintegrate the structures of opinion and break down patterns of behavior or information processing. They expose you to the idea that what you think you know isn't true. - Terence McKenna-

Psychedelics, the Magic Cure for Mental Disorders?

Around the world, millions of people suffer from mental illnesses However, prescribed treatments for these disorders have mixed results. Certain cases are even deemed not treatable. The psychedelics however prove that it can be treated better!

In the US treatments using a variety of substances are provided to conduct research. They include psilocybin MDMA (ecstasy), LSD along with ketamine, marijuana, and.

The rate of success of these treatments is evident, since 80percent of the participants are completely free of mental illnesses one year after the treatment.

Depressionen:

In studies conducted in clinical settings there has been evidence that LSD Psilocybin, LSD, and ketamine may be extremely beneficial over the long term affect on mood. Ketamine is even readily available US as a prescribed drug for depression.

The stories of people who have succeeded in fighting depression are so astonished that major newspapers like The New York Times, Time or The Guardian published the studies and the stories of those who were evidently healed of depression with psychedelics.

https://www.theguardian.com/society/20 12/jan/23/magic-mushrooms-psilocybin-depression-drug

http://healthland.time.com/2011/06/16/
magic-mushrooms-can-improve-
psychological-health-long-term/

http://www.nytimes.com/2010/04/12/sci
ence/12psychedelics.html?_r=1&

The psychedelics do not just help with depression, but also anxiety and post-traumatic condition, headaches in clusters fears of dying, and more.

On the website http://howtousepsychedelics.org , you can find a step-by-step treatment manual.

Additional information can be found on the home page on the website of the Multidisciplinary Association for Psychedelics research (MAPS). http://www.maps.org/research/psilo-lsd/

It's not an accident that this type of medicine is imposing its influence on the modern world. These herbal teachers are among of the best tools nature uses to communicate with humans. Their message is to increase consciousness in us as a defensive method to safeguard the sentient being that we are called Mother Earth. Iboga can be described as the tree that holds wisdom. Ayahuasca is the soul's wine. Together, they make up an entire, organic language that seeks warriors of the truth to communicate the message from Mother Earth. They call us to join them and communicate with us in a direct spiritual form, and they ask for our participation in the world or in the struggle to survive so we can restore the balance of our nature. -Dylan Charles-

Are Psychedelic Substances Addictive?

The concept of taking the term "drug" to combat the addiction to another substance appears incomprehensible to many.

However, there is a expanding research understanding to manage the effects of specific substances. The most promising drugs are psychoactive substances. These are the best suited for this job because they are mostly not toxic in the sense of therapeutic and do not trigger addiction. If handled in a wrong manner and/or in excess, psychedelics are known to create bad experiences, which act as a buffer to discourage the use of.

A lot of addictions serve as problem solvers, and they avoid the confrontation with the. The opposite is true for psychedelics as they trigger issues from the past that come to the surface and one has to face these issues.

Ibogaine, in particular, is believed to create a specific anti-addictive effect. Ibogaine's addictive properties were discovered accidentally through Howard

Lotsof in 1962, who was a heroin user in the moment.

When Lotsof consumed Ibogaine, he went on an exhausting 32-hour journey. When he finally woke up the next morning he discovered that it was not the same as when he used to take heroin. The experience was pivotal for the continuation of scientific and medical research.

Ibogaine's effect is not comparable to methadone that is being utilized extensively in the fight against addiction today. Methadone is a highly addicting opiate that is only the illegal substance that makes it legal. Ibogaine is a more profound influence on addiction as it functions in a variety of different ways.

The ibogaine molecule is in contact with a variety of receptors within the brain, yet in the same way, it is not a great affinity for them. This is among the reasons that school medicine is not addressing the issue and label Ibogaine as a "dirty drug". But, it also functions at a biochemical level since it is able to bring brain receptors back to the state prior to the addiction.

In addition, it could cause emotional daydreams that help users to confront the past issues on a different level.

Ibogaine can also trigger a long-lasting increase in a growth factor protein, also known as neurotrophic glial growth factor (GDNF). GDNF appears to play a significant part in the long-term anti-addiction effects of Ibogaine. Ibogaine is extremely lipophilic and is able to remain in tissues of the body for months at a stretch which can prolong this anti-addictive effect.

But ibogaine the most popular anti-drug psychedelic does not offer a 100% certainty that you will be free from addiction. However, it does provide an opportunity for those who want to change their behavior can achieve it. [1]

Recent studies have utilized Psilocybin to treat addiction to tobacco and alcohol. These are ongoing studies on policies using only small samples of random at present, however, the results are encouraging which is warranted. Of the four patients treated with psilocybin in the treatment of addiction to tobacco three were able to quit smoking for one year following treatment.

A recent study examined the effectiveness of psilocybin in treatment of alcohol dependence and found the significant abstinence over the long term of the participants (over 36 weeks) following treatment with psilocybin. It was not associated with any major adverse effects.

Conclusion:

Based on my studies and my own personal experiences the physical dependence on psychedelics is almost gone. In addition, the risk of addiction-related mental illness is practically non-existent.

The Pineal Gland - The Seed of the Soul

For a long time the pineal gland has been believed to function as an organ for out-of-sight perception, an opening to other dimensions like the third eye. In the past, it was lost to history, as scientists began to see that it was an organ that did not have any purpose, similar to the brain's cecum. The situation changed after the sleep hormone , melatonin was discovered.

As we learn more about the purpose of this gland step-by-step it is gaining significance in the present.

Researchers have discovered that, in addition to numerous hormonal functions the pineal gland may be the place where DMT is created and released.

The pineal gland is situated in the middle of our brain. According to some , it allows us to receive images and thoughts via telepathic communication.

It was first mentioned for the time in the writings by Pythagoras and Plato in which it describes as being a gateway into higher realms. [Urfeldforschung p. 69]

The pea-sized, roughly pea-sized gland is referred to as pineal epiphysis, glandular pineal, or third eye.

It's interesting that the pineal gland does not protected by the blood-brain barrier , and consequently, it isn't a part belonging to brains from a biological perspective.

In the present, the pineal gland is the subject of numerous legends and mysteries. Let's see the secrets we can discover below.

The eye is the source of light for the body. If your eyes are louder then your entire body will become light" Jesus -

Mythology

The gland of the pineal is frequently depicted by a pine cone, and is a major part of the sacred structures around the globe. The biggest sculpture made of the pine cone is located in a garden in the Vatican and at the foot of Pope Francis where a pine cone has been installed.

After reading this, I made an effort to look it up and went towards The Cologne Cathedral. In fact, I saw ornaments in the shape of pine cones at different places, so during your next trip, make sure to take an in-depth look.

Even in the more distant culture, this symbolism isn't a rare sight. To give several examples: If we examine Buddha sculptures, that spot between the eyebrows should not be ignored; it symbolizes the third eye, and the hair of Buddha often resembles an elongated pine cone.

A symbol of the third eye can be located in Islam. The sacred stone Kaaba is a tiny spot with a polished open edge; it appears like a horizontal third eye. Therefore, the Kaaba could also represent the pineal gland. Although Hindu gods are portrayed almost exclusively using a third eye and a lot of Hindus are still wearing this image today.

The most famous symbol of the pineal gland originates from Egypt It is an eye that is a representation of Horus. Horus's Eye of Horus is a prominent figure in the old Egyptian mythology, and at least in anatomical terms these similarities cannot be denied.

Left: Eye of Horus. Right: View through the brain, showing the pineal gland.

The pineal glands are often stylized and are represented with snakes that twine. These depict the energy flow through the spine and into the pineal gland, possibly activating its full capacity. This is known as Kundalini Energy.

Another example can be found on a rod dedicated Osiris. Egyptian god Osiris and can be seen in an art museum in Turin, Italy. Two snakes weave around the rod and place the heads of their snakes on pine cones located at the top of the rod.

It is quite remarkable it is that the exact same symbols is used in a variety of different cultures around the globe. Perhaps our societies aren't so different as we believe and it is possible that the rebirth of pineal glands could be the main factor that led to the development of a variety of different religions and cultures? We'll explore this issue once more in depth elsewhere.

Modern Research

Doctor. Rick Strassman was the first scientist to research what happens to the body when you take DMT with the permission by government officials of the US government.

This is a brief overview of the participants during the trials clinically: "To take a breath of this extremely potent substance has taken me beyond my imagination , and has overloaded the brain but the pure DMT injection through the vein could increase the effect to the unimaginable ... I am extremely proud of the courage and interest of the participants!"

Let's go on ...

Doctor. Rick Strassman conducted extensive research on impacts of DMT on human beings. Based on his findings the pineal gland acts as an open window to other aspects of our existence.

But, Strassman wasn't the only scientist who was able to study the pineal gland, and to report astonishing things. In the 17th century Rene Descartes claimed that human beings consist of two primary components: the body and the soul. The pineal gland as per Descartes is the connection between them. According to him the pineal gland can be associated with sensation imagination, memory, as well as the stimulation of bodily motions. The pineal gland is located deep within the cerebral cortex, it appears to be designed to transmit signals as per recent research findings similar to the retina of the retina of the eye. Researchers discovered that the gland was anatomically very as the eye since it contains the same light receptors, known as pinealocytes.

The light receptors are able to receive images that are visual and transmit them to different parts in the brain. The question is: what is the reason our bodies create an actual third eye , if there were no images to view? What are the sources of images from when we're dreaming or having an experience that is out of body or when a mental image is projected in our mind? Why should the pineal gland be at fault for a supernatural experience? (The Urfeld Research p. 76[The Urfeld Research p. 76]

S.S. Boconnier provides us with the answer by presenting a study from 2002. He found piezoelectric crystals made of apatite, calcite and magnetite within the pineal gland. The crystals of piezoelectrics can absorb electromagnetic waves, without electrical power. The nearby waves cause these crystals to vibrate, and they create sound. A radio operates exactly in the same manner.

Additionally, piezoelectric crystals are able to produce various quantities of light (photons) at a specific pressure, referred to as piezo luminescence.

We can clearly observe this principle of operation through an ignition source like a lighter. If a certain amount of tension is applied to the surface of the flint it creates a spark.

With this electromechanical-biological transmission mechanism, images and sounds could theoretically be generated directly in the pineal gland to be interpreted as internal visions of our brain.

Incredibly, DMT is a piezo-luminescent substance, similar to micro crystals. This brings us a significant step closer to unraveling the mysteries of DMT.

Of course, more study is required to better comprehend the way the pineal gland functions, but the knowledge that we have at hand gives us an amazing understanding. In the chapter"The Hidden Truth Behind the Fourth Dimension" I will go on exactly the subject and you will discover my view of the effects for the release of DMT in our brains and therefore, the perception of reality.

Dangers to the Pineal Gland and our Health:

Regarding our well-being the pineal gland has an important role because it is involved in a variety of vital hormonal processes within our body. A key hormone that is produced by the pineal gland , is sleep hormone, melatonin.

It is converted by Tryptophan, an amino acid serotonin before transforming into the hormone melatonin. Serotonin has a significant impact on our mood, and Melatonin is responsible for regulating the sleep- wake cycle.

Melatonin is a protein that can be produced in the dark , and suppressed by sunlight. It is also an antioxidant with a potent effect that shields the entire body from damage to cells. Additionally, melatonin has a particularly significant anti-aging effects.

A regular maintenance of the melatonin concentration reduces the rate of aging and results in a longer life duration.

Recent research has shown that in favorable conditions, the human body can to significantly age over 100 years. Melatonin may play an important part in this. The following figures could reveal to us the reason we don't get to this point in all instances.

Title: Melatonin production per age, green baby puberty, toddler lower at a higher age and a minimum in high-age Age (years)

It is evident that the level of melatonin declines dramatically with age.

So, if melatonin's role is essential for general health and wellbeing, then we can use these data to prove a significant connection between the production and concentration of melatonin within our bodies and the rise in the incidence of age-related diseases. To confirm this research on aging and hormones, William Regelson carried out a study that drew the attention of the world. To test his theory that the pineal gland acts as the real ',life clock" and that it is the "life clock," he carried out pancreas transplants on several lab mice. He also transplanted pineal glands of older animals to mice, and reversed the process.

The outcome is:

The mice for that no transplants were performed were able to attain an average of 720 days or 2 years. This is in line with the normal lifespan for these animals.

Contrary to this, the young mice, who had been given the pineal glands of their conspecifics older after 120 days only lasted 510 days in average.

In contrast, the older mice that had pineal glands of younger mice mouse, and then the 120-day-old mice aged 540 days had an average of 1020 days.

In interpreting these results it is important to remember that the findings of studies using laboratory mice can't be transferred to humans in a ratio of 1:1. According to their main assertion, however they affirm that the pineal gland generally speaking, plays very significant, perhaps even essential, part of the regulation of the aging process. 2. Regelson performed some more interesting experiments that all yielded the same result.

Fluoride: Distinctions and Facts

One of the main antagonists for the pineal gland the fluoride but there are a variety of fluoride.

There are a variety of fluoride, however I can only differentiate two. One is the fluorides that are classified as harmful, for instance: sodium fluoride (NaF) and potassium fluoride (KF) that also contain fluorine substances like

Hexafluorosilicic Acid (H_2SiF_6) sodium fluorosilicate ($Na_2[SiF_6[$) sodium monofluorophosphate (FNa_2O_3P) or ammonia silicon fluoride ((NH_4) $2SiF_6$).

On the other hand, there is the low liquid calcium fluoride (CaF_2) that is classified as non-toxic.

The water-insoluble fluoride, such as calcium fluoride is much less toxicity than the other fluorides discussed. [5]

The shocking fact is that the toxic fluorides, that are often referred to as sodium fluorides, are present in the food we eat everyday.

Sodium fluoride is a mixture of various heavy metals and chemicals, it is found in salt and is thus present in around the majority of our foods purchased from supermarkets.

It is present in toothpaste and mineral water too. The fluoridation of our foods is a huge problem, and if you are concerned for your pineal gland,, you must stay clear of it.

The problem lies in the fact that this gland itself isn't protected by the blood-brain-barrier, which means that the fluoride could easily connect to the crystals and then surround them with a thick mineral layer.

Doctors also make use of the calcified pineal gland during an MRI of the brain to assist in the direction of cancer detection.

It is also the one that has the highest concentrations of sodium fluoride within the body. It has been established that fluoride can affect converts tryptophan into serotonin and the melatonin. A dysfunctional pineal gland, resulted from the deposition of brain sand, and the fluoride-related calcium oxide, can significantly hinder the production of melatonin, and lead to serious diseases like cancer.

The Journal of Pineal Research published an important research on this subject, which reveals the variety of problems that can result from a calcified pineal gland.

There are numerous indications from the study to suggest that melatonin is a major factor in the emotional process and also in the processing and control of memory.

Melatonin levels that are low are frequently associated with schizophrenia and depression disorders. It is believed that 90% of schizophrenia sufferers are suffering from insomnia that is caused by the low level of melatonin.

Serotonin levels that are abnormal are thought to be the reason behind many illnesses too.

In addition, dyskinesia or Parkinson's disease. Also, epileptic seizures.

In this regard, an alarming statistic regarding the rate of calcification in the pineal gland is:

Africans: 5 - 15%

Asians: 15 - 25%

Europeans: 60 - 80% [6]

Most shocking is the effect of fluoride on human mental health.

Research has shown that over time, small quantities of fluoride slowly diminish the person's capacity to fight dominance.

Then, in German as well as Russian prisoner of prison camps during war, this information was employed to make prisoners stupid and eager to do their work". [7](From ,,The Biochemical Manipulation of Humanity" by David Rothscum)

I was skeptical about this for a long time however, I was proved not to be right, since as of April 2016, there were conducted 57 research studies looking at the connections between increased fluoridation and the human brain. The conclusion was that fifty of the 57 studies showed a clear link between fluoridation levels and decreased intelligence. [8]

Even if you don't think that fluoride is harmful to your body, be aware that there isn't a lack of fluoride!

Fluorides aren't essential trace elements, so they don't have to be added to our diet to ensure our health.

This is verified by a research study where mice were fed low-fluoride food for many generations. The mice were healthy even in their third generation. [9]

The inorganic or artificial sodium fluoride is the most poisonous protoplasm magnet which is 15 times stronger that arsenic." Dr. Charles A. Brush director of the Cambridge Medical Center in Massachusetts

Not only does fluoride have negative effects in the pineal gland. mercury (for instance amalgam fillings in dental procedures using amalgam) as well as alcohol, tobacco, caffeine as well as refined sugars may cause the pineal gland to calcify too. As we know, the micro crystals inside the pineal gland be exposed to electromagnetic radiation, which means that electromagnetic fields from external sources like power lines wifi radiation, cell phones HAARP, wifi etc. are major threats towards the pineal gland. Wireless Internet is now available in increasing numbers at no cost, yet we do not realize the risks that this technology poses. Pineal glands are organs sensitive to electromagnetic fields from outside and for in the long run, if we are in an environment that is harmful the pineal gland will not be able to achieve its maximum potential. [10]

I am Calcified - How Functional is my Pineal Gland?

It is important to know the function of your pineal gland functions.

To determine the function the pineal gland scientists perform the following tests.

The test isn't very long, so it is best to take it now.

All you have to do is shut your eyes and think of five colors randomly selected. If you can see an image in the mind's eye hold it for three seconds before moving onto your next colour. Try to imagine them as intensely as you can.

Can you see all of the colors clear and bright or was it all in black and white?

If you are able to be able to see all colors clearly the pineal gland is active. If you only saw the shades in white and black the pineal gland is not working or has diminished in its functions.

However, the inactive pineal glands can be activated, and tips for activation are discovered in the next section.

Tips to Activate the Pineal Gland

One of the most effective methods of activating the pineal gland is to meditate at the point that the inner peace settles and the body is relaxed and the pineal gland becomes well-supplemented with blood, just in the same way as it does at night. Take a deep breath and be aware of your breathing when you are in meditation. Focus on the part of the forehead in between your eyes. [9]

* Sleep in complete darkness. Total darkness stimulates melatonin production, ensuring a restful sleep. Make sure that all appliances are off.

A few tips A few tips: If you have to rise at late at night, but you don't want to disrupt your melatonin production it is recommended to make use of a candle or red-light bulb in place of the normal light. The typical light that comes from energy-saving bulbs operate in the frequency range that tells the body that it's the daytime. The body will then decrease Melatonin production as well as commence to shed cortisol. This would drastically decrease the chances of having sleeping soundly.

The practice of sun gazing can be a simple technique. It stimulates the brain and increases the health of nerve cells. It is as simple as looking at the sun at safe hours: either during the hour following sunrise or in the hour prior to sunset which is when there is minimal UV radiation. Start with 10 seconds , then every sunny day, add another 10 seconds. If there is cloud cover, don't add any more time.

* MF therapy provided by Dieter Broers

It is a must to avoid fluoride. Fluoride is found in drinking table salt, water, and toothpaste. To eliminate fluoride mixing chlorella and Spirulina algae performs an outstanding job since it binds and releases heavy metals.

Detox your body using a mineral with an excellent binding capacity to toxic substances (bentonite or zeolite, for example.). The toxins fixed by the earth can be eliminated as swiftly as is possible through the intestinal tract. Help your liver to be cleansed by using preparations such as milk thistle, the root of dandelion, turmeric and bitter substances like bitterstar or similar. Entlaste deine Leber mit Praparaten wie Mariendistel, Lowenzahnwurzel, Kurkuma, und Bitterstoffen wie Bitterstern o.a.

• Drink between 2 and 2.5 Liters of pure spring water each day, to ensure that a significant portion of the dissolved toxins will be eliminated by the kidneys too. Inhaling essential neroli oils stimulates the the pineal gland.

* Sing as frequently as you can, since the vibrations produced during this process stimulate the pineal gland.

Ayahuasca - Wine of the Soul

The ayahuasca drink is an original mixture of the harmaline-rich Ayahuasca liana banisteriopsis Caapi as well as the chacruna leaves that contain DMT (Psychotria Vidridis). Harmaline acts as an MAO inhibitor. It inhibits releases of natural enzyme monoamine oxide (MAO). The MAO usually breaks down the visionary-psychedelic drug DMT (= N, N-dimethyltryptamine) even before it can enter the central nervous system via the blood-brain barrier. Only through this combination of active ingredients can the potion show its consciousness-expanding effect and trigger visions. [1]

Jeremy Narby comments on this complex dish in the book The Cosmic Serpent with the words:

One has to wonder how people living in a primitive world lacking any understanding of physiology or chemistry could arrive at this conclusion:"Alkaloid gets activated when it is stimulated by monoamine-oxidase inhibitor." 2.

Translated from various indigenous languages Ayahuasca refers to something similar to the tendril of souls bitter medicine, medicinal plant as well as the cure. [1]

In Spanish the word shamans is "ayahuasqueros". The shaman draws his healing power shamanic through the knowledge he gains through his frequent or every day consumption of Ayahuasca.

As time passes Ayahuasqueros acquire an amazing amount of knowledge about dealing with Ayahuasca. There are rumors of shamans believed to have consumed the brew each day for more than 25 years. [1]

Within those who are Shipibo Indians from Peru, Ayahuasca is believed to be a healing agent for mind and body. Ayahuasca, on the other hand, is believed to have a profound psychological effect on the mind that manifests by mystical visions and inexplicably vivid travels into other realms. However the drink has a powerful detoxifying effect as well as vomiting and sudden diarrhea. remove the body of numerous pathogens.

I think that this substance is responsible for supreme shamanic ecstasy. It is also responsible for awakening, as well as to enter the "clear the light that is death"." Christian Ratsch

Knowledge on Another Level:

Ayahuasca is a powerful herb that can help you relax the shaman can see spirits who reside present in animals, plants mountain ranges, and streams and then can make contact with them.

From them, he gains the information about their own innermost being.

As a result, he discovers the significance of each animal and plant every single mushroom, and recognizes that each species is unique and has its place within the life cycle.

Could this be the case?

As such, ayahuasca is not just a treatment, but the method of gaining wisdom from other dimensions of the mind.

And if we accept the tales of people of the Amazon region, Ayahuasca can do exactly what it says.

They claimed that they were firm and authentic that they acquired their vast knowledge from hallucinations induced by psychoactive plants.

This is why it is among other reasons that the many names of places in the Ayahuasqueros' areas originate from their visions.

A different example is curare. Curare is a plant with a paralyzing effect on muscles. toxin used to treat blowpipes. It has an established purpose, which is to kill animals living in trees, without causing permanent harm on the flesh. Furthermore, it should be able to relax muscles which means that the animal is able to let go from the tree and sinks onto the floor.

What is the likelihood for the native people of Brazil to have picked specifically these from 80.000 plants found within the

Amazon region, given that a variety of plants must be combined and need to be cooked for 72 hours to get the desired result?

According to them, ayahuasca is a rational being which provides knowledge and power when all rules and regulations regarding nutrition are taken into consideration.

It's almost not necessary to point out that these individuals consider their dreams to be like we treat our own reality.

Can Ayahuasca Cure Cancer?

We're not aware of the cancer-causing effects of ayahuasca. But I found some studies and reports that may provide us with some details.

Eduardo E. Schenberg, who is employed by the University of So Paulo in Brazil is of the opinion that healing qualities of ayahuasca merit the attention of scientists particularly in relation to cancer. In an article that was published in Sage Open Medicine, Schenberg writes:

,,There is ample evidence that the active ingredients of ayahuasca, especially DMT (NN-dimethyltryptamine) and harmine, in some cell cultures used for cancer research and in biochemical processes used in cancer treatment both in vitro and in vivo, have important positive effects.

White-man-medicine can make you feel great at first , but then unhappy later. Native-American medicine can make people feel awful at first but then good later. -Anonymous-

One Man's Experience of Cancer in addition to Ayahuasca:

Schenberg's research examines a number of articles about a possible cure for cancer using Ayahuasca. One of them is the amazing tale that was told by Donald M. Topping, published in 1998 by MAPS (Multidisciplinary Association of Psychological Research).

Topping recounts his experience of healing through ayahuasca and his personal experiences during the ceremonies. According to him, Western doctors basically condemned him to death, therefore Topping searched for alternative ways to heal and came across the ayahuasca. His cancer was completely eradicated.

This Schenberg study also includes the findings of Robert Forte, who accompanied two cancer patients during Ayahuasca-based sessions as well as clinical studies. A prostate cancer patient was treated with surgery, which reduced the level of his PSA (a prostate-specific antigen that is used for detecting cancer) to zero. However, 10 years later, his PSA increased again. Another patient was diagnosed with advanced ovarian cancer that had metastasis. Both patients were evaluated clinically prior to and after the use of ayahuasca and both showed significant improvement.

A Canadian doctor in Canada, Gabor Mate, tried the use of ayahuasca for cancer patients. He concluded that ayahuasca is not a cure universally effective, however he believes that when used when used in the right setting and with the appropriate support Ayahuasca could be a crucial part of cancer treatment and healing process. He currently assists cancer patients by providing Ayahuasca, under the guidance of the indigenous Peruvian Ayahuasqueros".

DMT -- Trip Report - Journey to another reality

DMT Trip Report of a Shaman

In the followingparagraphs, I'll present to you a travel report which impressed me particularly. Patricio Dominguez was an South American shaman and was one of the volunteers of Rick Strassman's clinic DMT studies.

Patricio Dominguez

The location where this experiment was conducted was a medical facility located in New Mexico. I picked this report due to the fact that it provides the reader with an extremely clear picture of a high dose DMT experience.

I was especially impressed by the way he conveys his feelings during an excursion.

To make this story more empathetic, I was comfortable to share my thoughts and interpret the facial expressions and body language from Patricio Dominguez. He then describes his experience through the experiment. Enjoy reading.

Experimental Tests using high doses of DMT

Patricio Dominguez:

"[Makes deliberate gestures] substance flows through your body at unimaginable speed. The sound in your head rises dramatically and you can feel the sound of the flowing water and an extremely high-pitched sound. It is easy to believe that in a loud environment there is no way to hear a loud sound however there is a distinct high pitch that is clearly heard.

Then there's the journey ... Yes, I think that the word "trip" is an appropriate word.

Then , the journey begins, and you're moving across time and space, and the surroundings are racing over you just as if you were in Warp Speed on Star Trek since suddenly everything comes to you at an incredible speed.

Your thoughts suddenly don't come in a rather slow pace as they do in the past, just like when you're thinking of something, and your thoughts are gradually shifting to new thoughts, or old thoughts slowly receding to the background, etc.

[visually exuberant and strongly gesticulating[excitedly and clearly gesticulating

Your thoughts are reverberating at incredible speed.

A thought occurs, it is smashed into your mind, you attempt to take it in and then a new one appears, and it's gone. Then another thought pops up followed by the nextone, and so on it's a matter of time before the thoughts aren't only thoughts, but are actually that are very big, and on top of the fact that images pop up in a high rate, far which is too fast to process at the same time, and the speed only is increasing. Then you begin to think: Oh this is too fast, just a more and I'll not remain pace with this speed. The images and data will appear at such a rapid pace that I'll get lost."

It can get to the level where information is just moving by, far larger than the mind is able to manage The result is the brain acts like a computer operating in overloaded state, and it goes down. Similar to that, click".

Your mind has gone, but that's only the first step. humans are a complex being, and we also have different layer (energy bodies) that we could be able to describe as human. The next thing you observe is that you've got an emotional mind. it's now just pure emotions . Things begin to overwhelm you. And immediately your emotions begin to take over you that they begin to collapse.

After having been through the various layers, you realise that "I are just my pure essence".

That moment, something deep and deep inside you is saying ...

You are dying "...

In the midst of all this information, an extremely clear thought comes into my mind and says, "I knew this would happen! I'm headed to the hospital and taking part in this study and someone cheated me with the wrong substance , and poisoned me, those insane doctors. The fact that I died in the hospital by a doctor it's a pity." But now, I'm dying. The layers of my humanness are beginning to fall off until eventually, somewhere you reach the final layer. I'm not able to say precisely what it is but it's the final layer that defines your identity as an individual human being.

His voice becomes gentle and slow] And there's no any longer a human being. it's not something you're able to recognize, you don't know whether you're an animal, mineral, a vegetable or something else but there's one thing you're certain about: [raises handIt is clear that you are no any longer a human being. He seems extremely touched. Everything that made you human being has gone.

Thoughts, emotions, emotions awareness all fell away completely from you , step by step.

[collapsed emotionallyThen you're what the texts of mystical literature have always tried to explain the pure consciousness that is that tiny spark of your identity. It's not an identity at all It's a state of consciousness.

The only thing that you know is that you're here! You don't know who is happening to you, and you do not know the place you are in however, you are there.

Very vivid, but the cost you pay for it is extremely high. In the process taking off all the human layers it's possible to feel a response with a cry. Like the baby. I did at the moment I lost my humanity.

[Seems lost in thought for a while, but then remembers the emotional connection[Seems lost in thought for a moment, remembers the emotional touch

It was my life as a for so long, but the more layers were removed the more I was crying and cried in absolute pain. I passed away however, I wanted to be human. I didn't realize how wonderful being person until the day I realized it in this present moment. you doubt that it's only temporary, you think that "I'll never become a human again," and there was an immense sadness for each layer that I lost, a tremendous sorrow ...

Then I reached the final stage of this journey and all geometric shapes like mandalas and mandalas as well as the bright lights went away ...

The smile returns his lips] Then I came across the second thing. There exists a consciousness or intelligence somewhere, or even something known as the creator and that the vast majority of people don't come to know the creator (even if they are emotionally involved) and certainly don't wish to visit him after hearing about how to go there it's not an pleasant journey".

Then you encounter the creator and it's not what you've read about in the ancient texts of mystical religion.

It is the creator who of the universe is ...

The excitement swells across his face]
broad, tall and comes in a variety of
appearances. This flash of consciousness
suggested is that it was linked to the
creator and I realized I was component of
the creator. This was then imprinted in
stone, that I was part of him. That implies
that I am also the maker, or at the very
least an atom that is his universal material.
[Happily excited]

It's even more because, when I realized
that I was component of the man, I could
identify the part I played which is
something which captivates me. In my
time as an shaman, I was able to study
numerous divine manifestations, and
gods, the great wisdom, and mythical
creatures also. As I found my place within
the nature created by God, I was able to
even tell what I was prior to that, I had a
face , and an identity of my own it was like
one of the beings I've read about

previously. I'm not going to discuss about it too much there are a few things that I have to remain private with myself. "In all likelihood, I found the identity of who I am. It turned out I was a very special person.

Okay, let me introduce an interesting fact. While I was in the realm of the creator and realized my identity as the Creator I realized that the DMT was losing its effectiveness. Now, something was happening. The creator I was to move on What could the Creator do? He designed a universe in which we could return to our normal lives.

[gesticulating] Step one by one, I set out to design a world which I would like to live in, and at the same time, I made my body as well as the physical world I'll return to. As I created my memories, I returned, and I made the world from my memories. I then created the world exactly the same the way it was before I had left. The experience made me a nostalgic person and I put things together the way I did since I had missed the experience so many times. Therefore, I made the universe exactly the way it was. Boom! With my eyes shut, I recreated the scene from the hospital in which the patient awokeI awoke and asked for the blindfold taken off of my eyes.

[Thoughtful] I must diverge a bit.

Being in union with God there is no concept of time. There is not even a precise term for space. There is just being.

As I returned home, with the sensation of time moving at a rapid pace I felt like I was in a solitary state for at least a thousand years. 1000 years perhaps more, but I'm not sure it was difficult to comprehend the events that were happening.

Then, when I returned to my body, and wanted to ask if they could remove my blindfold, the memories of what transpired was finally brought in my mind: I was in the hospital, and the doctors had murdered me. But then I realized it was actually a hospital and I thought, [laughingat the thought, "Oh, I are incredible, and in some way the hospital kept my around all the time, possibly for research reasons or maybe they thought I'll be able to come out of the coma in time. I can not believe they kept it for that long." Then I wondered if there might still be a distant relative of mine out there, perhaps a great-great-grandchild or so, or if my name was still somewhere in the books, or if there were any books at all? ...

The Breakthrough The First Real Experience with DMT

Prior to my first DMT journey, I drank DMT in very small doses.

Since I created the product myself I wasn't sure the possibility of it causing damage to the body.

Thus, I was cautious. I purchased an ordinary cigar and advised one my closest friends to look after me in the event of an incident. I was ecstatic because I didn't know what could befall me. However, I was not worried as I wanted to discover what was in store for me at the end of my tunnel. Therefore I started adding the crystals of white over the tobacco, while thinking about how to prepare myself. I took a deep breath before lighting the mixture. I took a little swig and then held it for a few seconds inside the lungs to see the way my body responded. After the initial analysis when I left my eyes closed. I didn't feel any internal discomfort, but I heard a low buzzing noise that was becoming more louder. The environment around me also seemed to have changed slightly. I could tell that the colors were slightly brighter and the surroundings blurrier than normal. It was a good thing, I thought. the first time I made my own DMT was okay and I decided to take another shot.

This time I took a more powerful hit, while letting the smoke remain in my lungs for a little longer than it did before and the effects began right away.

The sound that was reminiscent of an old CRT television got more intense and I was somewhat odd. I shut my eyes and with astonishing clarity I was able to see an incredible mandala-like shape. It was stunning and I felt as if I was inside a room. I was able to look at the left and right. My eyes opened, and the reality appeared to be blurred. Then I shut my eyes once more and gazed at the stunning mandala until the illusion gradually diminished.

Overall, this event lasted about 2 minutes.

After my trip, I realized that I required more information. That's how I discovered Terence McKenna.

And I remember the shock I felt at the time Terence McKenna described a great mandala-like creature he names Chrysanthemum when he presented his lecture because that's exactly what I saw.

The following weeks, I was able to only think of one thing: DMT! So I gathered as much information as I could and began to plan my next adventure.

I'm sure I understand why Terence McKenna says you have to take the third one due to the fact that on the next occasion I couldn't bring me to consider taking the 3rd one. I believed that the second was enough however, that wasn't the situation. Then I saw this mandala-like creature that changed my perception and also several other things. However, it was quite disappointing given that it was the most potent hallucinogenic drug known to man. Thus, taking the third one was my ultimate target for the next time. That's how it got me into my breakthrough!

Since the result did not satisfy my expectations from the things I thought and read I lost some admiration for the substance. But I'm not going to make the same mistake again! You could think that the subject felt this disrespect and I, with my self-confidence high and confidence, slapped me in the face , which put me back to ground.

The following occurred:

To achieve the objective, "This time, I'll achieve the breakthrough" I was able to extract an additional amount of DMT. In this case, I did not use pipes but constructed something larger. In my home country it's commonly referred to as a "bucket" in English the same way as it is "Gravity Bong".

I grabbed the 1.5-liter bottle and cut the bottom, placed an aluminum foil head on top, and then placed the bottle into an empty bucket of water.

If you place something in the head and ignite it, pulling it up from the bottle pulls all the smoke to the 1.5-liter bottle. All you need to do is to remove the head and take smoke from the bottle. That's the fundamental idea behind.

It's done and dusted. When I took my first puff in the bottle it was obvious I knew this was sufficient (it was approximately 20 mg per head, and it didn't completely went away). I didn't even manage to hold the smoke in my lungs, considering the speed at which the effects started to kick in. I couldn't even exhale the smoke from my lungs and then fall onto the couch after it started to kick into.

The beeping sound, which typically began slow, was not noticeable to me. The sound was loud immediately, akin to an impact when something large is thrown down. Then I felt the sensation of being on a roller-coaster that was soaring through space at around 1,000 kilometers/hour. It was dark, yet vibrant things flew past me and my thoughts were whirling at a rapid pace. The majority of them were negative thoughts, and they caused me to feel quite uncomfortable.

After around 2 minutes of the rollercoaster, and all the thoughts and data coming at meat a rapid pace, I became certain that I would be dead by at any moment. But I couldn't stop being an human. I was unable to continue. I tried to reconnect with my body, but wasn't a success since the roller coaster kept going around and around. However, at some point it stopped. The room was dark, and there was something in the room. I couldn't see it but I could hear a voice which told me to take a look. In the same time it was a rising rainbow made up of tiny balls were visible from bottom to right. Each ball was distinct colors. The structure was not too complicated, however the spectrum of colors was breathtaking. Then, I heard the voice over and over, and the same rainbow was visible on the other side, only with slight differences in color. I was able to unwind my mind for a while however I wanted to return. I thought about people whom I was close with and I was sad.

I've not lost anyone whom I was extremely close to me. However, I'm sure I understand the feeling of never meet a loved one ever again. The feeling I experienced was completely real.

I was so happy when I realized the effect was diminishing. I tried to relax my eyes, however, there was an overlap in reality. The room was entirely different in the initial moments, but I had to force myself not to shut my eyes since I didn't want to return there. I was desperate to be human! In terms of time, it appeared to last for about 15 minutes, however in reality it took just three minutes. I laid on my couch and let what I felt settle into. I shrugged my shoulders for about 5 minutes. I escaped with only a "boah," followed by a five-minute laughter, after that, I was forced to cry for a couple of minutes. In the report written by Patricio Dominguez of emotional and information throughout the trip was too much for the short amount of time. Following the excursion, I was physically and emotionally overwhelmed.

After 15 minutes, I was fully restored.

And I was so delighted to see my mother back soon after.

The event changed everything throughout my entire life. I was convinced that what I witnessed didn't originate from my imagination; everything seemed so real.

Terence McKenna mentioned that DMT does not affect the judgement mechanism of the mind. Thisis something I am able to verify. It's like you are altering the reality of reality.

The moment you start smoking DMT it is like jumping on the train of interdimensional reality toward the unknown. The dose determines how long the journey will stretch. From my experience, it's not even possible to have a conversation that is level with someone who's never had this trip.

This is an Experience Report of a Different Kind.

A participant in Rick Strassman's DMT test series experienced the most shocking experience, totally different from the previous two reports.

The following excerpt is from the book "DMT the Molecule of Consciousness" by Rick Strassman.

[Ken] sat down around the 5 minute mark, but then he grinned and shaken his head. After a couple of minutes, he retracted the blindfold and looked straight ahead. His pupils were still dilation and Laura and I sat still and waited for the pupils to fall further. In the span of 14 minutes, he produced an uncooperative however, he did make an impression of calm and began to talk.

Two crocodiles were in my chest. They raped me and crushed my chest. me sexually. I was unsure how I would get through that. In the beginning, I thought that I was dreaming, and then I experienced an unreal experience. But then I realized this was actually taking place.

I was happy that it was a test day and that we had not utilized the rectal probe.

The eyes swelled with tears however he didn't weep.

It sounds horrible."

It was horrible. I've never felt this much fear in my entire life. I was tempted to ask to hold your hands however, I was smashed down to the point that I was unable to speak or move. My God"

To the Source of Life and Back Again. DMT Trip Report that includes 80 mg DMT along with Passion Flower Extract (MAO Inhibitor).

It's true that I've had a few experiences with DMT which included one or the other breakthrough experiences. This is why I decided to increase it just to a little bit and even exceed my previous dose limit that was 60 milligrams.

In the beginning, I'm trying to create a delicious DMT-Changa mixture, which will be able to fit into a small head. It was a success and, naturally. As my Changa dry, I took a deep internal journey and did some meditation. I was overwhelmed with admiration and respect, which was not the case previous trips. I knew it would be a long-distance trip. So, I thought at least twice before I decide, however, my scholarly nature was able to shout , "Yes you can!"

Like every other time I started purifying my body and surroundings by using Palo Santo, looked at the Changa and it was dry, began building my pipe, and then completely filled my head with the Changa and listened to Indian meditation music. I breathed deeply and sat down on my sofa and placed the hookah in my mouth. A little doubt was raised - it isn't it? Do this now!

Then, with a quick thought I ignited the Changa and went on my way. Inhale and quickly remove the pipe and put it back in the sink. It's a shame, getting it out of the way is already a struggle and I'm very hot. hot. When something grips my neck. I lie on my back and shut my eyes. I do this every time I do my usual closing of my eyes because there's visible light passing through my eyes. With eyes completely closed, I'm able to let myself relax more while the physical effects get intensified. But back to the issue. I'm on the couch and everything on my body begins to shake.

The notion of time does not have any meaning. It was like a sudden warmth, and in front of my eyes, the usual kaleidoscope image that is becoming increasingly

131

vibrant gradually begins to shift and rotate like an array. I did not feel myself within my home or as a person In reality, I just felt. It's difficult to define; I'll come back to this in the future. The kaleidoscope's matrix is getting more and more vibrant, and is moving in a more chaotic manner. It suddenly screams and flushes, and I fly through what I'll call the light corridor, the size of a tunnel that is derived from the kaleidoscope perspective. Then I'm flying through space and time according to my impression, it's like I'm carried through a black hole which is not black at all. It's stunningly vibrant, in shades that aren't in any color chart in the world. I could describe it however I don't know the way to describe it. There was a flush , and I was suddenly sucked into blackness I looked up and saw colors and everything was sputtering out of something. It is possible that I was shot by these bubbly things, and would slowly sink to the ground , or more precisely I don't see any ground. I can only see colors beneath me. I then sink, however, as I am falling I realize that I do not have a physical body. In reality, I've seen nothing of myself. I could only see the surroundings. I felt, however and the feeling was awe-inspiring and difficult to describe. However, I'll give it test. It was like I felt pure energy as if were power. I'm using the word "electricity" due to the fact that I've experienced an electric shock prior to that, and the sensation I experienced was close to. It did not harm me, rather it did the opposite. You suddenly realize that you are energy in all its purest form and you feel an euphoria as well as peace and salvation in its most pure shape.

It was like I was standing right in front of the colourful world. At least it doesn't feel as if I'm falling. Then I glance around and find it difficult to concentrate on any thing.

Everything is so vibrant and it's a wonderful feeling. At once, I can see the shape of an apple or a torus appearing before me, similar to the magnetic field of the earth. Looking back, initially I couldn't even comprehend the vision. The torus literally exploded with all the knowledge one could learn about biology, chemistry and the physics class, and much more that I am unable to explain because there aren't words to describe it. It was then clear that I don't have a physical body . And since I did not, as I expected to be a part of a realm of trolls and fairies, I needed to process the first. A sudden feeling told the me everything would be fine I needed to let go, and it was wonderful to discover it there. Then I realized I had come out of the torus right in front of me the torus. I felt an immediate warm sensation within me. I'm not sure how but I knew that the torus right in my view appeared to be the center of everything that is life.

It is a divine thing pure in action. After having a better understanding of all this, I was now eager to know more about it and headed toward the Torus with the intent of smacking into it. A sudden voice is telling me yet again, but with no voice. It is difficult to explain, that it was not my moment and that I must return slowly. I was not sure what this meant. What should I do, I'm exactly where I need to be and it's gorgeous. Then again, return to where you are. At that point I saw two cats wailing from further from me, but I cannot pinpoint where the whining originated.

In front of me, suddenly I saw a red dot appears. This may sound odd to some, but this particular point has been accompanied by me in my DMT and has been identified to be my dog who died. Then I followed the line again, it led me through a vast and vibrant world of unfathomable patterns and patterns, until the edge which was where all the colorful things were behind me, and before me was the darkest black and absolutely nothing other than that. At that point, the cat's whine got more and more louder, and I was also conscious of the music.

In my gut, I knew that I'm going to have to return to finish my sentence. The light bulb starts to blink as I say goodbye to him and say , until the next visit, Berti. The point grows larger and then says goodbye to me as well and says that we will meet again soon.

My time was now and I was supposed to leave. I was supposed to go in the direction of familiar sounds and feelings. I glance at my pet to inquire or point and again, but where should I go?

There's nothing around me. It is then that I realize I am something that has appeared from nowhere. If I'm in a state of no where and I'm not going anywhere, I must be something. I did not take a long time to think about it, took a deep breath, knowing there was nothing to take and took an immense leap into the void. I feel the rush of vitality slowly fades away and I drop from the bright world to an unrecognizable black world. Then, suddenly, a squeak and a whoosh. My eyes open, and I'm sitting on my couchwith my two cats sitting on my head, looking happy that I have finally met them. They didn't leave immediately. One thing I want to say to you, dear readers, I've not taken this much breath. That felt as if I took my first breaths. Following that, I consumed the equivalent of one Liter of fluid since I was feeling very thirsty. In addition I was feeling like a the newborn I was. I realized that my body was at a world in which everything we could but cannot imagine is actually created. The journey has altered my thought patterns. From being a meat-eater to a vegetarian I had never thought of and then did the trick. A week later, after the trip, and where I'm writing this article today, I am still able to see the things changed for me. Like I said I've experienced several things through DMT I've worked in various different areas, but what encountered this time was the most profound experience one can experience and feel. In just a few days I was able piece together a few elements that revealed the place I was and what I experienced there. I hope you liked my report. I'd like to make sure that I will not repeat it. This kind of thing is unique and difficult to comprehend for everybody, or wanting to escape from the world or accept its powerful nature is difficult.

Abstract Interpretations of a DMT Experience

On the Internet There are a myriad of theories of an DMT experience that can be found. Below are eight imaginative interpretations. Which of them sounds the like the most plausible option to you? you decide. I wrote my own interpretation in the chapter , "The Hidden Truth Behind the Fourth Dimension". Certain of these interpretations such as the experience itself are quite absurd, however the author suggests that each concept must be considered because the truth may be not just stranger than we imagine however, it is also more terrifying than we imagine. Take the interpretations as thinking experiments, that could be further developed as you wish.

1.) There aren't any beings (intelligent beings) These are subjective hallucinations. The DMT experience is extremely intriguing, but there aren't any entities that exist beyond us. The possibility of this would reduce DMT down to an absolute minimum level and transform it into a brain-based art that can create the most stunning and amazing things inside our brains. [1]

2.) DMT provides access to an alternate or higher level of reality alternative to the one that exists in reality as inhabited by independent intelligent entities. [1]

3.) DMT enables the perception of processes on a levels of the atomic or cellular. DMT smokers have the ability to look into the neural network of cells within the brain and even the interactions between molecules. It could be even an understanding of the quantum mechanics on the subatomic or atomic levels. [1]

4.) DMT is a neurotransmitter that comes from a very old brain region. When DMT is absorbed into our body and causes it to trigger the reptilian* part of our brain to assume the control of our mind, and the state is then considered to be a journey. [1]

5) Intelligent, non-human species evolved into humans through genetically altering the existing primate population, and then retreating and left biochemical ways for interaction with them. The psychoedelic tryptamines act as chemical keys which activate specific programs in the human brain. They were deliberately inserted by the alien species. [1]

6.) The world that DMT gives access is the realm made up of dead. The entities are souls , or people who have passed away that maintain some form of communication and life. The realm of dead souls widely accepted by societies and cultures not tied to the materialistic view of the world and is now available to DMT. [1]

*Reptilian Brain *Reptilian Brain Brain Stem is most ancient and most deep part that the human brain has. It was developed around the 500 millions of years during the process of evolution. It is home to all the vital regions which constitute the essential requirements to sustain the existence of every vertebrate. In reptiles, this region is the brain's entire area which is why it's called.

7) The imaginative beings are creatures that have been able to master the art of traveling through time. But not in a manner that allows materialization, but the way that they are able the ability to interact with other conscious entities similar to us. [1]

8.) The creatures are probes of alien species released to other contact species that can alter their nervous systems in the way that communication could occur. [1]

So long as we're still unable to comprehend the entire process that we experience, we should not look to determine the objective credibility of this experience, instead, we should take advantage of the subjective impact on these experience.

What can we gain out of these events? What can we learn from these experiences? What can we learn from these experiences to effect transformation in ourselves and the world? [1]

Holotropic Breathing

Holotropic breathing is a powerful of a self-experience that is often highly effective and psychotherapy technique that works on states of altered awareness. It's likely to trigger a discharge of DMT.

It is said that Dr. Rick Strassman even associates the breath of holotropics with psychedelic experience that is spontaneous. Every person, using this technique can trigger the sensation of a DMT experience with no external sources. The name itself suggests that the holotropic breathing technique is a specific breathing technique that permits the user to experience different state of mind.

Effect

It is believed that holotropic breathing can have powerful, "opening" effect. This makes it an addition to conventional psychotherapy to treat depression.

Used ,,blockages". People who have practiced holotropic breath have reported an entry into the spiritual realm together with higher understanding and healing.

In Holotropic breathing, breathing becomes intense and rapid for a period of 30 to 60 minutes.

Professor. Callaway, of the University of Kuopio, Finland, expressed the fascinating hypothesis that hyperventilation can raise your body's level of dimethyltryptamine. This is an assumption based on the fact that huge amounts of the N-methyltransferase enzyme is present inside the mammals' lungs that, when released, produces dimethyltryptamine by combining with the endogenous tryptamine.

Holotropic Breathing Instructions

In Holotropic breathing, there's no specific guideline, other than the suggestion to breathe more deeply and faster than usual. It is essential to remain totally relaxed. Most of the time, your body will establish its own rhythm within 15 to 20 minutes, but until that point, it is essential to focus on breathing.

Step by Step

1.) Deep breaths and full-on deep breathing.

Inhale through your nose and take a breath out of the mouth. It's not just about taking deep breaths. You should take the most deep breath you can. In the event that you do take a very deep breath, the entire air will be blown out. This can feel strange however, you must be sure to hold your deep breath and fast rate for a short period of time. If you start to feel dizzy take a break for a few minutes and remain in the present. Focus on breathing and block out any other thoughts. One way to clear your thoughts is to visualize the thoughts of clouds. Don't focus on the clouds; instead, observe them while you focus on your breathing. Once you've achieved the art of taking deep breathing, you're well-prepared to take the next step.

2) Continuous, ,,circular" breathing. Breathing should be performed in a way so that there aren't any gaps between breaths. The breathing should not cease at any time. If lung capacity has attained while you inhale, switch your breathing around and begin breathing out. If your lungs are empty after exhaling, begin breathing in again. This will create a breathing pattern where you are always inhaling or exhale, forming the cycle of breathing.

3.) Speedier than usual - it is recommended to breathe more quickly than you usually do. However, you shouldn't breath so quickly that it causes tension in your body. Your body, and in particular your lungs should be relaxed to ensure that your breathing pattern can be maintained for a long time without becoming exhausted. If you notice that your body is tight you should slow down your breathing to a certain extent, but you should maintain the volume of your breathing. Within 15 to 20 minutes, your body will adapt to the breathing.

Hints:

It's not a problem to alter your breathing method. If you prefer breathing by your nostrils or mouth continuously it's fine provided you're totally relaxed.

A complete breath through the mouth is a great way to let out more emotions.

Recumbent positions are generally preferable. It is recommended to keep a trip sitter on your side.

The more frequently you engage in this method, the more easy it will be to attain higher levels of awareness. This is similar to advanced meditation practices and psychic experiences.

Soul Journey Breathing Technique

Here's a method I came across on (eve-rave.ch) (eve-rave.ch), a Swiss site for drug forums: "I wanted to show my own method to stimulate the body's own DMT.

I've not been to the sleep lab, but I've observed some interesting aspects regarding my lifestyle. I'd like to briefly discuss the subject here.

I would like to invite the maximum number of people to take this on, so that we can discuss the subject more effectively.

It's true that I didn't take part in it too often, but I've observed that the technique works best when you do it in the evening prior to going to sleep. The best way to do it is challenge your body to the limits and then exhaust it completely by doing lots of sports and exercises. I typically do around 50 pushups before I am unable to do it anymore. In the next few minutes, I hyperventilate to the point that I that I inhale and exhale in a way that is exaggerated. You look totally insane, but other people wouldn't keep from laughing.

When you inhale lift your arms then drop them when you exhale like you were inflating your ribcage.

It is best to imagine jumping out of a plane , without having a parachute, and then just waiting for the moment of impact.

Dwell on it !!! Take a deep breath and inhale deep, breathe for as long as possible and then, when you exhale then inhale just as deeply and slowly as you did previously. Repeat this for a few minutes. then you'll notice that the sensation of tingling on your skin is evident and you will experience an intense concentration capability despite the fatigue. You now have plenty of oxygen in the blood, and your mind is in a condition of crisis. You should try to keep this state of mind.

Lay down on your bed, in a dark bedroom. Then, do the reverse. Relax!

It is best to lay straight on your back and rest your neck firmly on pillows to ensure that your head is slightly tucked behind you, much like when you go to the hairdresser.

It is recommended to keep hands straight, or keep them placed on your stomachs.

And then breathe between breaths to get lots of oxygen to the bloodstream, and you're able to lie in bed.

Then relax! Relax and lay flat.

Once or twice, you'll experience a change of a frantic breathing, and calm.

Try to sleep.

While I'm to sleep, an odd sensation is felt over me, and my body begins to vibrate. At first I believe I'm asleep. I'm trying to get up at this moment, but then I realize I'm awake, but not moving.

I'm paralyzed, and I feel an intense sense of terror. It's difficult to define the aftermath. My soul is separated from my body, which seems to me to be the most plausible scenario.

I've flown over many continents, and I'm sure. Then, you can relax in a soap bubble or floating across the room however you'd like.

The fear that my soul will never come back into my body is a smack in the face. If that was true, then I'd likely be in a state of numbness indefinitely, completely void of consciousness.

A different time I was able to experience the process of forming a triad (three-element unit) along with two human souls, an accumulator of souls.

We were one entity and had three souls. It was similar to the way you think of in the Collective Unconscious by C.G. Young.

The present day, it could occur to me at any time but I'm unable to anticipate it precisely. Similar to that, it occurs to me between 2 and 5 times per year in a single year. Two times I couldn't attend school the following day because my mind was completely unfocused.

I think it's an result of DMT However, it could also be exactly it is an OBE (out of body experience). [1]

Changa - Smokable Ayahuasca

After the appearance of the smokeable Ayahuascas a new era began to emerge known as the "Changanautik"! It was invented by Julian Palmer" and awed Changa the globe and became an integral part of the psychoedelic scene.

Palmer came up with the name "Changa" as a result of an Ayahuasca ceremony in response to his query regarding a suitable Name for his blend of herbal smoke. Based on Palmer, Changa is an evolution of Ayahausca as well as an

an independent tool that can be used for psychedelic, therapeutic, healing, and for ritual use. Another benefit of Changa is the ease of use to take it.

It is easy to smoke in a bong or pipe without paying too any attention to whether the DMT is properly vaporized. It's even feasible to use Changa in the joint. Particularly for DMT newbies is this an exciting option since you have the most complete control over the experience.

If you believe that smoking Changa is just a more effective method to bang away" then I'm going to have be the first to diss you. The psychedelic chemicals are in the mix,

that are, according to Terence McKenna said, ,,only disguised as drugs however, in reality they are the keys to different levels of consciousness and reality.

These substances may assist us in exploring areas that are not yet explored by modern science.

What is Changa?

Changa is a mixture of smoke made up of psychoactive plants.

Changa is also known as a smokeable ayahuasca. The most common draught horse instances is N-N-DMT. It's rare to find 5-Meo-DMT. Then the addition of a plant acts as a MAO inhibitor e.g.

Banisteriopsis caapi or Mullein. Because the MAO-inhibiting action of plants is a subject of debate the use of harmaline is often applied for the flower in its free base form. [1]

Different combinations of smoke can produce different effects. The addition of Salvia Divinorum enhances the hallucinogenic effects. In addition, adding Damiana enhances the effects. comfortable and sexually stimulating. Users are saying they feel that Changa is a much more convenient method of smoking DMT. Furthermore the effects are extended up to 5 to 10 minutes due to the MAO inhibitors. [2]

The most famous Changa blends made by Julian Palmers

Original recipe:

Ayahuasca Android:

70% Caapi - 30% Chaliponga

Palmers originals, no. 1:

40% Ayahuasca liana (Banisteriopsis caapi leaves)

20 20% of Peppermint (Mentha piperita)

20% Mullein (Verbascum densiflorum)

10% Passionflower (Passiflora incarnata)

10% Blue Lotus (Nyphaea caerulea)

Dream include:

30 percent Ayahuasca Liana (Banisteriopsis caapi - leaves and Bark)

30 30 percent Aztec Dream Aztec Dream (Calea zacatechichi - leaves, buds and stems prior to fruiting)

20% Heimia salicifolia (sinicuichi)

10% Justicia pectoralis

10% Damiana (Turnera diffusa)

Changa classic:

30 30 Banisteriopsis caapi (leaves)

20% Damiana (Turnera diffusia)

20% Passionflower (Pissiflora incarnata)

20 percent peppermint (Mentha piperita)

10% Blue Lotus

The Mekong:

50% Blue Lotus

50% passionflower

Electric Sheep:

50% Blue Lotus

50% Dream grass (Calea zacatechichi)

Minty Blast:

40% Caapi

35% Pfefferminz

25% Konigskerze

Original Blends of Changa (without DMT) according to Julian Palmer.

original recipe you can find on the website ,,das-dritte-auge.com/changa-blends".   If you request, the Changa-Blends will be shipped to all countries in the globe. All you need be doing is to add the Freebase DMT into the herb mix and then the original Changa-Blend is now ready.

I suspect that this substance is the one responsible in the final shamanic experience, for awakening, and for getting into the 'clear light of the afterlife'. ,,(Christian Ratsch 1998)

Changa - Do it yourself

The following explanation of how to create Changa does not constitute an offer to engage in the crime. This description is intended for information only.

Ratio DMT in plants

Julian Palmer (inventor of Changa) suggests the following: There are two factors to think about when making Changa 1. Which herbs should I employ and 2. What is the strength of my blend be?

The most important aspect is the proportion to DMT and the herb mix. Mixing ratios determine the amount of Changa is required to smoke in order to attain the desired effects. A low DMT to herbal mix ratio is not recommended because you will need to consume more in order to reach the peak. A mixture that is too strong is suitable for experienced DMT users, but it is not recommended for novices to take a dose. However, each Changa blend is based on the preferences and desires of the user. When selecting a mix, it is best to rely on your intuition. However, experimenting with various combinations can be interesting and assist you in finding the most enjoyable blend for you.

A ratio of 1:1 (Freebase DMT Herbal Content) is an effective mix for the average consumer and can be the catalyst for a breakthrough quickly.

A 2:3 ratio (2 components Freebase DMT: three herbal parts) is slightly weaker as it gives the mix more influence over the experience.

If you are planning to create the Changa blend using this formula to determine the ratio of blend.

To help you understand this better, Here are two example calculations:

Example 1: make use of the Freebase DMT equivalent of 2 grams in an amount of 2:3 (2 part Freebase DMT for 3 natural parts)

In the example 1, we require 3 grams of herbal mix!

Example 2. In this case we'll make use of 1 gram Freebase DMT in 1:1 percentage (1 portion Freebase DMT for one herb component).

In this example 2 you will require 1 gram of herb mixture!

After you have calculated the quantity of herb matter using the formula, you are able to begin weighing. Cut the plant material until it is in the shape you'd like to smoke in the future. Then weigh how much Freebase DMT you require for the mixing ratio.

The next step is that you will need to dissolve the Freebase DMT. (use approximately 40 ml of solvent for 1 grams of DMT).

Solvents that are suitable are, specifically:

Ethyl alcohol (ethanol)

Acetone: In the drugstores you can purchase acetone to remove nail polish. Purely it is also available it in hardware stores.

Always remember the safety precautions regarding the extraction of psychoactive substances.

For for a container, it's recommended to use a smaller ceramic bowl. It must be small to ensure you can ensure that your plant materials are fully coated with the solvent containing DMT.

The mixture of herbs and solvent (acetone)

Add the herb mix to the dissolving DMT and mix well. If needed you need to add more solvent to ensure that all the ingredients are coated. It's now time to rest. Put your bowl inside a calm area for a couple of days. The acetone will take about 4 days before it dissolves without leaving any residue and the herbs are fully dried. Once everything is dried take a weight of the DMT mix of herbs. Weight of herbs ought to have been a part of the weight of Freebase DMT.

Changa After 4 days

It's done! Simply and in just two steps, you've achieved Changa. :)

Always take care to treat DMT with reverence and appreciate the fact that you be able to hold this amazing substance in your possession. Use the knowledge you gain from it to the benefit of the world.

Yopo - Snuff Tobacco of the Gods

Yopo ritual

Yopo is an psychedelic and psychoactive snuff made from the bark and seeds from the Yopo plant (Anandenanthera peregrina, and Anandenanthera colubrina). The powder is introduced into the nasal passages through tubes and induces psychedelic reactions due to close contact of the mucous membrane of the nose.

The reports of experience have described multi-dimensional visions which manifest in a variety of ways. Common experiences include communicating with phantoms, rebirth dreams and spiritual connection to the natural world (ego dying).

The effects of Yopo begins after 30-60 seconds and lasts approximately 15 minutes. To increase the effectiveness it is recommended that another MAO inhibitor (beta-carboline) is consumed during various occasions. Beta-carbolines also provide an effect of purification on the body. This could cause severe physical symptoms, such as diarrhea and vomiting.

To be able to eat the seeds and get the psychedelic effects, mature seeds should first be lightly roast. Then , they are crushed to the finest gray-green powder.

Dosage:

The dosage minimum is 1 grams of seeds. The dosage is always suggested for application of the nasal spray.

An gradual increase in dosage is suggested. [1]

Iboga - The Tree of Knowledge

Ibogaine is an alkaloid isolated that is extracted from the root bark of the Tabernathe Iboga (marigold). It is a species of plant that has been used for a long time to treat and heal spiritually within Central Africa. In low doses it acts in a way to provide a remedy natural to combat fatigue. However, at high doses, it can be an effective psychoactive drug that has hallucinogenic effects and can affect all five senses. It is frequently employed in ceremonies of the past to induce a death-rebirth sensation and also to connect to the Divine.

It is for this reason that it is also revered as an oblation plant.

Tabernanthe Iboga

Ibogaine, which is used to treat drug addiction, is believed to have an anti-addictive effect. The latest western treatments are studying the effects of ibogaine on mental illnesses with remarkable results. Ibogaine's anti-addictive qualities were discovered through chance through Howard Lotsof in 1962, who was an addict to heroin during the period. The details of this are in the chapter on Suppression of Spirituality.

African people take a bite of the root to remain awake for several days as well as to connect with the ghosts of their ancestors. It is believed to be to be the spiritual leader of the human race.

Effect:

If you're considering taking Ibogaine, I recommend you find out more. High-dose trips could last for up to 24 hours. Additionally Ibogaine is a MAO inhibitor. This is why I suggest taking a small dose at the beginning. For more information, visit erowid.org.

Legal status:

In Germany Ibogaine is not covered by the BtMG. In July 2014 it was decided by the ECJ declared that the substances and preparations that are not considered narcotics and that are intended for intoxication purposes are not medical products, and consequently, the production and placement in the market for this reason is not prohibited by The Pharmaceuticals Act. [4]

Foods that help you unlock your spiritual Potential Tips for your everyday life

The pineal gland provides the brain's primary source of energy. We have discussed in the past chapters, the gateway to greater mental power. This is a sign of greater creativity, more motivation, better mood and other unique capacities. It is believed that the opening of our pineal gland is in general an opening in our minds, which is why we should make the pineal gland a higher importance.

Unfortunately, our western culture is exactly in an opposite direction. No matter what It is now time to start to take our spiritual and spiritual growth in your own hands. If we wish to attain this, it's essential to incorporate this knowledge in our everyday lives. This is why I'll provide you with some tips to help you do this.

Foods do not just contribute to the calcification of the pineal gland. They may also help to reactivate it. An ideal way to start your day could be the combination with Passionflower, and St. John's wort.

But, you shouldn't overdose your daily intake of 3-4 cups.

Passionflower can be described as an MAO inhibitor, meaning it stops certain neurotransmitters like Serotonin, from being blocked. MAO inhibitors can be found in a wide variety of foods, like chocolate, with large amounts of cocoa. This is why chocolate boosts our spirits. MAO inhibitors can have powerful effects upon our moods that they're prescribed as antidepressants in addition.

The most potent plant that can boost spirits is Rhodiola. Rhodiola boosts the levels of serotonin by about 30 percent and aids in the transfer of 5-HTP to the brain. It is also an efficient MAO inhibitor.

DMT is created in small amounts by the body in the course of metabolism, but it is activated by monoamine oxidase. When we consume small amounts of MAO inhibitors, our body's DMT is retained in the bloodstream for longer. In the same way the low-tyramine diet must be followed by the consumption of MAO inhibitors since certain compounds that are consumed in the diet cannot longer be degraded and result in a toxic reaction.

To increase the effects of the pineal gland you could also consume small doses daily of ayahuasca. You can prepare Ayahuasca by yourself using Banisteriopsis Caapi as well as Psychotria Viridis using Orange juice. This Banisteriopsis Caapi contains MAO inhibitors as well as Psychotria Viridis has DMT. A teaspoon of a mild broth at the beginning of your day can be a good start. In larger doses, ayahuasca can cause powerful effects, such as visions and a change in the perception. In smaller doses, it only awakens the brain and increases the mood, creativity and the ability to see.

Another ingredient is melatonin.

Melatonin is well-known for its anti-aging and antioxidant properties. It is also known for its capacity to help promote healthy sleep patterns and to protect us from electrosmog.

If people begin taking supplementation with melatonin, many feel more empathy and feelings that result in better relations between family members and friends.

I highly recommend the book "Extremely Dosed" Written by Jeff T. Bowles, in which he discusses the ways that melatonin and other compounds can reverse or even cure numerous illnesses. In Germany there is a prescription required for melatonin , and it is not permitted as a nutritional supplement. On the other hand, on the internet you can purchase it from countries that are neighboring. Foods that contain melatonin are Montmorency cherry, wheatgrass along with barley grass. Festuca arundinacea grass contains the highest amount of melatonin in a plant.

Research has proven that yoga and meditation enhance the production of melatonin. Simple breathing exercises and yoga over some months could trigger substantial changes to the level of melatonin.

It is crucial to help our pineal gland to function biologically in our daily lives to discover our way back to a higher level of spirituality and back to us.

Everyone has the potential to be higher spiritual power however only a handful of people are willing to release this power. The book you read is an excellent start but the practical wisdom is much more valuable than the theory.

If you've read this book, you're probably not done at this point. You're only at the beginning of your long and arduous journey, towards your most optimum state of being.

Psycedelics: a path to gain insight? Part 1

It is believed that American psychotherapist William James claims that humans are able to trigger changes in their behavior in two ways. One of them is the "normal" learning model that is where the changes occur step-by-step. There is a distinct type of learning that is commonly called a conversion experience quantum change, or the moment of illumination.

In this case you suddenly experience a profound behavioral change takes place in response to a particular moment or a particular knowledge or experience. The question that is most intriguing is: can the use of psychedelic drugs can actually trigger a sort of awakening moment that creates a radical shift to our everyday lives?

The quest for answers takes us on a different adventure, leading to a completely new perception of these elements.

But, before we go further into the topic we must first define what exactly is meant by the term "enlightenment".

", "enlightenment," also called illumination is a type of spiritual experience which

One may get the impression that their everyday consciousness has been elevated and that he is experiencing a unique perception of an attained, holistic reality."

In modern times"enlightenment" culture, the term "enlightenment" generally refers to sudden understanding or revelation.

The first step is to ask What is an insight or a concept occur?

Recent neuroscientific research addresses the issue, and some amazing results are revealed. But it's all step by step:

Our current understanding of science indicates that our brain is home to around 8 billion neuron. Together, they make up a complex network, which is made up of billions of neuronal connections. Our Neurons are stimulated, for instance by our thoughts or even by unconscious stimulation. But, they also can be activated in a spontaneous manner. Some are active cyclically in specific patterns, and some are activated only a short time before turning off or are activated when input comes from other neurons is received.

It is in the right order. Even if we think of nothing or are asleep, it produces neural activity a frequency that can be measured by EEG (electroencephalography). The frequency created by neural activity creates a brainwave. However, we actually have multiple brainwaves due to the fact that neurons perform distinct activity in different areas in our brain. This is how different brainwaves can be created simultaneously.

The greater the amount of activity, the greater the frequency. However, the lower the activity less frequency. This is why we have discovered that brain waves don't appear in a uniform frequency, but instead are a mixture of different frequencies. To make the essential connections clear, let's look an in-depth look at the purpose of brainwaves.

6:30 a.m The alarm goes off and you awake from a sleeping. You get up and dress to start your day. From here, until a few seconds later

In the rest of the day, you'll likely spend the majority of the day in the predominant brainwave state Also known as "Beta".

The state of consciousness is associated to the range of frequencies of 12 to 30 Hz (Some researchers limit beta to 25 Hz). When the state is that there are various types of focus, commitment and intense mental activities. In the lower end of Beta brainwaves (12 -15 Hz) you are able to define your mood.

as passive or relaxed (example such as getting stuck in traffic, chatting browsing the Internet browse).

As a cat standing on the other side of an open hole for mice Relaxed, but always eager to leap. In the middle of Beta (16 -22 Hz) one is described as being highly active (example being active and analytical problem-solving). The higher band of Beta (23 -30 Hz) corresponds to highly sophisticated thinking as well as the integration of fresh experiences, and excitement (example creativity in problem-solving).

If someone is awake, but in a relaxed state then their EEG wave is classified as "Alpha" that is between 8-12 Hz. A characteristic of this kind of consciousness is if you are dreaming during the day , or when you are in a calm, unengaged state while watching television. The subsequent EEG wave is known as the "Theta" brainwave and ranges between 4-8 Hz. The behavioral characteristics include relaxed and a light sleep state. Theta is also known as a brainwave state in deep hypnosis or during deep meditation.

The most slow-moving kind of EEG wave is related to deep sleep, also known as "Delta" and ranges between 0.5 to 4 Hz. Only meditation experts who are experienced can achieve the state of deep meditation.

If we can assign the four types of brainwaves (Beta Alpha, Beta Theta as well as Delta) to the state of consciousness that we experience in our daily lives, then this result in the hypothesis that a higher frequency is associated with higher concentration, greater attention and more precise cognitive skills.

However an increased brainwave frequency can reduce the cognitive capacity of our brains to the point at which we are unable to comprehend complicated information anymore.

In the end, we can conclude that a person with 12 Hz is in a "daydreaming" state. The state is at 22 Hz , highly involved" while at 30 Hz, he, they are capable of solving complex and imaginative tasks. However, is there something beyond this "Beta" state, perhaps an extremely enhanced mental processing capacity?

In 2009, there was a study in the journal "Current Directions in Psychological Science" was titled, "The Aha! Moment, the brain's cognitive neuroscience of insight ,,. This research was based upon the study of the neural correlators (factors in mutual relations) in the moment of sudden understanding of problem-solving times that can be interpreted to be an "insight" or "Aha!" moment. EEG devices as well as (fMRI) functional magnetic resonance imaging were utilized to study how much frequency (Hz) and regions within the brain activated during these times.

The study found that insight or solutions, also known as "Aha!" Moments, correlates with bursts of Gamma waves (40 Hz). Gamma waves" are brainwaves that occur of 30 Hz.

Gamma waves aren't easy to spot due to their small magnitude. This is why they couldn't be studied more thoroughly up until 1970. Gamma waves are classified as 30 Hz or more. Here's an excerpt from Brain World Magazine from the study of 2009: "A third second prior to the subject reached the answer we commissioned an avalanche of Gamma waves. A flash of Gamma wave waves occurred

in the right hemisphere the brain, that is involved in problem-solving as well as association processing. The Gamma activity shows a cluster of neurons that bind to each other for the very first time the brain. This creates an entirely new neural

Network route. This is the start of a brand new concept!

Following the Gamma-wave rash, a new concept is revealed in

our minds and rate it as an Aha-moment that is unique to us."

Additionally, Kounios and Beeman noticed the slower release of Alpha wave activity in the visual cortex on the right - the area of the brain which helps us perceive our surroundings and is observed just prior to the onset of Gamma waves. This result is a surprise and indicates that our brain is calming the neurons of this region to decrease visual distraction as is the case in daily routine, in which we shut our eyes in order to greater focus on one thing. This could lead to new knowledge faster to our minds.

A study published in the year 2008 was a research study entitled "Deconstructing Insight" was released, with similar findings: "We detected significant Gamma waves (40-48 Hz) in the parieto-occipital area. It is thought to be an intense state of selective attention that either leads to a mental deadlock as well as a valid solution, based on the intensity in these Gamma waves. This way, fresh spontaneous solutions are possible as part of a treatment for a problem. This finding is fascinating and appears to indicate that certain parts in the brain get purposefully relaxed (brainwave decreases) to produce Gamma waves later.